Lifestyle Makeover for Diabetics

Lifestyle Makeover for Diabetics

GEORGE TOHME

LIFESTYLE MAKEOVER PRESS

Copyright © 2007 by George Tohme

All rights reserved. Except where indicated, no part of this book may be reproduced in any form without written permission from the publisher and/or the author.

ISBN-13: 978-0-9791215-0-0
ISBN-10: 0-9791215-0-7

Library of Congress Control Number: 2006939228

Published in the United States of America by:

>Lifestyle Makeover Press
>2911 Turtle Creek Blvd
>Suite 300
>Dallas, TX 75219

Printed in the United States of America

Dedication

I dedicate this guide to all those who've supported and assisted me during the writing of this work. My brother and sister's love and support have been pivotal during this process. My beloved mother has been the driving force throughout and until the completion of this guide. My father's wisdom and advice to professionally stick to my field of expertise lives with me; this has pushed me to reconsider my options and move forward with this guide. God bless and rest his soul.

Special thanks to Chantal who helped me type part of this guide and kept pushing me to meet its completion deadline. Also, I thank the support and love of my family the Walkers and friends in West Virginia. I value the support of my friends in Dallas, especially Joe and Sandy, for helping me in the editing process; they have done a terrific job. Monnie and Glenda's final touch has been very valuable.

I would like to acknowledge a tragedy that deeply marked my extended family and me before this work saw its completion. That is the loss of close relatives Fuad and his older sister Suzy as cancer claimed their lives almost one year from each other; they were in their forties. We grew up together; we were next-door neighbors and best friends. They are missed.

Crucial was the inspiration I received from the friendly people in the numerous towns and cities in Texas that I visited while I was working as a traveling pharmacist and where this guide came to fruition (namely Dallas, Fort Worth, Jasper and San Angelo).

Finally, I dedicate this guide to you, the readers, as I believe in my heart that this guide will make a difference in your health and your life.

Foreword

It is not that global warming is not an important matter but the opposite is true. Our planet is the concern of all of us. All nations of this earth should come together for solutions otherwise the future of our planet can be troublesome. However, I will leave this issue to be addressed by professionals in this field and policy makers. But right now there is an urgent major threat that has been inflicting tremendous harm, claiming endless lives and causing major debilitations to countless others in our society and all over the world. This threat is avoidable and it is called Uncontrolled Diabetes.

The inception of this guide started as a vague idea when I was 13 or 14 years old, growing up as an overweight kid. I was overweight the first 17 years of my life, due to overeating, binging and absolute inactivity. I am well too familiar with the scars that such a physical state can leave on anyone's feelings, emotions, and self-confidence. Ill informed I lost about 85 pounds, within a couple years of my 17th birthday, by unconventional methods such as starvation and attempting every "diet" available.

In the process, I became a veteran at riding the roller coaster of emotional peaks and valleys of alternating feelings of success, guilt and failure. For the last two decades, I have persistently searched and researched, informing myself of the ideal way to lose weight permanently without dieting or deprivation.

After completing my pharmacy degree in Pittsburgh, Pennsylvania, and after years of being engaged in targeted specializations in preventable and lifestyle-related chronic diseases such as diabetes, high blood pressure, high cholesterol and obesity, my persistence paid off and led me to the answer.

The answer is, making favorable lifestyle choices. I share my revealing findings in Action: Step 4 of this guide. Had I not lost that weight initially and later maintained that loss by making favorable and balanced lifestyle choices, as I describe in this guide, I would have become much more obese and would have very likely acquired diabetes, and might now be battling its deadly complications.

What's in This Guide?

This is a comprehensive guide for people who have or are at risk for diabetes. The helpful and eye-opening instructions found herein will help with the daily challenges and choices a diabetic has to make. This guide also serves as a helpful resource for healthcare professionals, supplementing the materials they offer their patients to read and follow. All information in this guide is based on the most recent research and recommendations of the World Health Organization, US health organizations and academic institutions such as The American Diabetes Association.

This guide contains the following crucial 5 Action Steps for ultimate diabetes control. Read and apply these 5 easy steps and prevent avoidable deadly complications. A must-read, quick-reference section is found at the end of each Step (or chapter).

The 5 Action Steps are:

1. Understanding diabetes

2. Knowing your diabetes medications

3. Monitoring of crucial parameters such as your sugar, blood pressure, cholesterol and others. Learn about treatment options for cholesterol and blood pressure. Learn about what deadly complications you can prevent

4. Learning to make favorable lifestyle choices and losing weight permanently by building new good habits, eating balanced meals and engaging in regular activity

5. Learning about stress relief

And a special section about:

- Boosting your sexual health regardless of age and gender

Contents in Detail

Introduction 17

Action Step 1: Understanding Diabetes 21
- How Is Diabetes Affecting and Impacting Our Society? 21
- What Is Diabetes? 23
- How Many Types of Diabetes Are There? 24
- Identification of Those Who Are Diabetic But Have Not Yet Been
  Diagnosed and Those Who Are Pre-Diabetic 27
- **What You Absolutely Must Know at a Glance from Action Step 1** 29

Action Step 2: Get to Know Your Diabetes Medications 31
- Critical Signs of Hypoglycemia (Or Low Blood Sugar Attack) 35
- The Various Classes of Medications Available to Treat Diabetes 36
- Insulin 36
- Proper Injection Procedure and Mixing of Insulin 40
- Insulin Storage 41
- Insulin Pump 41
- Exubera 42
- Very Important Tips about Insulin 43
- Oral Medications to Treat Type 2 Diabetes 44
- Byetta 51
- Symlin 52
- The Importance of Taking Aspirin or Other Blood-Thinning Medications 54
- Ask for Generic Drugs…How to Bargain for the Best Medication Prices
  And Tips on Finding Cheaper Drugs 54
- Which Pharmacy Should You Choose? 56
- **What You Absolutely Must Know at a Glance from Action Step 2** 57

**Action Step 3: The Vital Importance of MONITORING Your Sugar, Cholesterol,
Blood Pressure and Feet; Treatment of Cholesterol and Blood Pressure;
What Complications Can You Prevent?** 59

Diabetes Complications 59
- Potential, Debilitating and Life-Threatening Complications of Diabetes 59
- The Harsh New Reality for Cedrick, Who Did Not Take His Condition Seriously 60

Monitoring 62
- Imagine You Are the Captain of a Boat in the Atlantic Ocean
  Without Navigation Gear 62

- Janet's Story Represents Millions of People with Diabetes: People Whose Condition Goes Unnoticed and Undiagnosed, and Who Quietly Suffer from Having Their Condition Slide Dangerously Out of Control 64
- Matching Janet with a Blood Glucose Monitor 66
- Telling Janet about Proper Blood-Drawing Techniques and Instructions On How to Minimize Pain 67
- Alternative Pricking Sites 68
- Important Lancing and Skin-Conditioning Tips 69
- Matching a Monitor with Your Specific Needs 70
- Janet's Inquiries 71
- "How High or Low Should My Sugar Level Be, and Why Is It So Important to Keep It There?" 71
- **The Compass Table of the Various Crucial Parameters that EVERY Diabetic MUST Know and Monitor in Order to Navigate to Safety** **72**
- "What Is 'A1C' and How Relevant Is It to My Diabetes Control?" Janet Asks 74
- "Why Is It So Important for Me to Check My Feet DAILY?" 75
- The Story of a Diabetic Employee Who Comes Limping From a Foot Ulcer to the Pharmacy 76

Cholesterol 79
- How Important is Cholesterol Control, What Are the New Recommended Cholesterol Levels, and What Medications Are Available to Treat High Cholesterol? 79
- Which Cholesterol Medications Are Available and What You Should Know about Them 81

Blood Pressure 90
- How Can Blood Pressure Be Controlled in Someone Who Has Diabetes? And What Is the Ideal Blood Pressure Reading? 90
- Proper Blood Pressure Monitoring Technique and Frequency of Measurement 92
- Here Follows the Story of Tyrone, Who Monitors His Blood Pressure ONLY at Every Doctor Visit, and the Danger That Created for Him 92
- Here Follows the Story of Ricardo, Who Had a Near-Stroke-Level Blood Pressure Reading and Was Near Collapse 94
- Selecting a Blood Pressure Monitor and Cuff Size 95
- What Is a Normal Resting Pulse 99
- The Several Classes of Blood Pressure Medications that Are Ideal For People Who Have Diabetes 100
- **What You Absolutely Must Know at a Glance from Action Step 3** **111**

Action Step 4: Lifestyle Choices: Learn to Make Favorable Lifestyle Choices; Learn How to Build New Good Habits; Make Favorable Food and Activity Choices; Lose Weight Permanently without Ever Dieting Again 113

Favorable Lifestyle Choices 113
- The Rewards to You, the Diabetic, If You Continues to Persistently Make Favorable Lifestyle Choices 113

Contents in Detail

- The Story of Wanda's Son Who Is Diabetic and Bakes Cookies
  And Eats Them in Large Quantities..115
- Here Is the Story of a Man Who Is Diabetic, Overweight and a Smoker
  Who "Doesn't Have Time" to Increase His Activity Level!!!................................116
- The Success Story of an 82-Year-Old Man Who Had Diabetes
  Under Control for 30 Years..117
- Alarming OBESITY Statistics! No Relief in Sight Yet..122
- Health Risks of Obesity..123
- The Good News..124
- Lisa Wants an Over-the-Counter Diet Pill Recommendation..............................125
- The Media Shoving Ridiculously "Thin" Models in Our Faces
  As Symbols of "Good Health"..126
- Chris, an Overweight Pharmacy Technician, Wonders Why
  He Cannot Lose Weight..127
- Identifying Barriers and Finding Solutions with Favorable Lifestyle Choices...128

Learn How to Build New Good Habits...129
- The 3 Habits that Will Transform Your Health and Life..129
- Unlock the Secrets of How to Develop New and Favorable Habits
  And Regain Unlimited Control Over Your Life and Health................................134
- What Is a Habit?..134
- John Doe's Current Habits: A Typical "Eat, Sit and Smoke
  Like There Is No Tomorrow" Kind of Day...135
- Try This at Home—Simple Proof that Anyone Can Learn a Good
  New Habit and Unlearn a Bad One at the Same Time.......................................139
- John Doe's Attempt to Have a Lifestyle Makeover..140
- The Common Actions of People Who Lost Weight and Kept It Off Permanently........146
- The Process of Learning and Unlearning a Habit and How Any of Us Can Adapt......146
- **The Spandex Phenomenon**..**148**
- Build the Foundation First and Learn How to Fish...148
- Never Feel Guilty Again...150
- Do We Need Willpower to Have Good Health?...150
- The Story of Toya Who Is Diabetic and Frustrated with "Low-Carb Diets"......152

Food Choices...157
- Lose Weight and Keep It Off by Making Food Choices as Follows.....................157
- What Are CARBOHYDRATES..159
- Unlocking the Puzzle of How the Excess Sugar and Food You Eat
  Ends Up As Fat under Your Skin..159
- Glycemic Index..161
- Carb Counting...161
- Simple Carbs..162
- Breaking the Hunger Cycle "Code"..162
- Complex / High Fiber Carbs...164
- Proven Benefits of Selecting Foods High in Fiber and Low in Sugar..................165

- **How to Get 35 Grams of Fiber Daily and Lose
  An Additional 250 Calories Daily**..**165**
- Try This at Home to Visually Witness the Impact that Foods with High
  Or Low Sugar Content Have on Your Blood Sugar Levels.. 166
- Sugar Alcohols as Sweetners 166
- "Net Carb" Count 168
- Deciphering "Low Carb Diets" 168
- Fats 170
- Proteins 174
- Become a Nutrition Label Reader 175

Meal Structure Blueprint for All People Including Diabetics................................ 177
- **PORTION SIZES (AN AVERAGE SIZE ROUND PLATE)** **178**
- **The Meal Blueprint** **181**
- Delicious Cooking Methods Other than Frying 185
- **List A**: Favorable Food Choices from All Food Categories...to Be Consumed
  As Discussed in "The Meal Blueprint" 186
- **List B**: These Are Less Favorable Choices of All Food Groups) 193
- General Food Selection Tips 197
- How to Assess the Portion Sizes of Food Recipes Which Contain
  A Number of Food Groups 199
- Meal Makeovers When Eating Out 200
- Keeping a Daily Food Log 206

Activity 206
- Making Balanced Activity Choices 206
- The Miraculous Benefits of an Active Lifestyle 208
- Common Excuses Why People Choose to Remain Sedentary 208
- How Anyone Can Make Over His or Her Current Sedentary Lifestyle
  And Make the Transition to an Active Lifestyle: Do it Now
  And Permanently Lose 10 to 15 Pounds a Year 210
- The Invaluable Use of a Pedometer 211
- Tips to Raise Your Daily Activity Level at Work, at Home and while Shopping 212
- **The 4-Foot Rule** **213**
- The Crucial Importance of Scheduling about 30 Minutes
  Of Brisk Walking 3-5 Times a Week 213
- What Is a Reasonable Approach to Progression in the Amount
  And Duration of the Activity You Choose? 214
- The Benefits of the 5-Minute Warm-Up at the Beginning
  Of Your Chosen Activity 215
- The Benefit of the Last 5-Minute Cool-Down Period 216
- How Fast Should You Go During that Scheduled Activity? The "Talk Test" 216
- Interval Movement Cycles: A Major Powerful Weight-Loss Booster 217
- The Revealing Benefits of Choosing One Progression Criteria at a Time 218
- The Feeling-Good Factor 220
- Why Is It Essential to Include Variety in Your Chosen Activities? 220

Contents in Detail

- The Fun Factor...220
- A Variety of Activity Choices to Include in Your Scheduled
  Activity Session on Different Days...221
- Always Stick to the Basics...222
- What About Jogging, Racquetball, Intensive Training and Team Sports?..............223
- Activity Log...224
- Safety Tips 224
- Proper Gear for Your Activity Sessions 224
- The Importance of Water Replenishment and Hydration 225
- Tips on Staying Active while Having Physical Challenges
  and Leg Neuropathic Pain..226
- If You Are in a Wheelchair...227
- What to Remember from All the Prior Information in This Activity Section.............227

Permanent Weight Loss...228
- Do We Burn More Calories at Rest or When We Move Around?.........................228
- Quick Tips on How Anyone Can Start Immediately Losing Weight
  And Keep It Off for Life...230
- "I Don't Know Why I Am Not Losing Weight"..232
- "I Hit a Plateau and Stopped Losing Weight after I Have Been
  Doing Well—What Should I Do?"...234
- **What You Absolutely Must Know at a Glance from Action Step 4 ....235**

Action Step 5: Stress Relief and Management 237
- Some Real Worries and How People Generally Deal with Them 238
- What Are Favorable Ways to Deal with Major Stresses?..239
- Major Stress Busters that You Can Start Practicing Right Now 241
- **What You Absolutely Must Know at a Glance from Action Step 5 ....244**

A Word about ALCOHOL..245

Women and Men: BOOST YOUR SEXUAL HEALTH AT ANY AGE...................249
- The Arousal Process and the Problems that Could Affect It 249
- Common Medications that Cause Sexual Dysfunction 250
- The Benefits of a Healthy Sexual Life...252
- Libido Booster for Men and Women in Three Easy Steps 252

Women 253
- What Treatments Are Available for Sexual Dysfunction in Women?.....................253
- Pregnancy, Birth Control, Vaginal Infections and Women Who Have Diabetes 255

Men..258
- What Treatments Are Available for Sexual Dysfunction in Men?..........................258
- Premature Ejaculation 261
- Add a Spark and Boost Your Sexual Life..262

Valuable Web Sites...270

Introduction

Do you have Diabetes and don't know it? Are you at risk of having diabetes and can avoid it? On page 28, you will find a list of criteria to determine whether you may have diabetes and should be tested. People who are overweight and have any of the criteria listed, but have not yet been diagnosed with diabetes, can benefit from the recommendations in **Action Step 4: Making Favorable Lifestyle Choices**. This information will give you the tools to gain permanent control of your weight and health and avoid developing diabetes, as well as other diseases.

Are you a smoker?

If you are a smoker, refer to **"Stop Smoking Today,"** my smoking cessation guide, and quit right away! Keep trying because smoking, as you know, is a deadly habit. It destroys people in the prime of life. Smoking expedites and worsens diabetes complications, and it makes you an easy target for other grave health threats, including artery disease, heart disease, debilitating or fatal strokes and heart attacks.

You will start healing only twenty minutes after your last cigarette, so please don't wait; quit today! The real and grave threats will not just go away, and the pain and anguish of poor health will get you sooner than you think, unless you quit. Don't wait. Quit now. Your loved ones will appreciate your presence, and you will shortly feel that you have become *much* healthier. You *can* do it.

This guide can be a lifesaver. Any person with diabetes or predisposed to having it can benefit significantly by reading this guide and applying the tips listed herein. People risk damage to their precious vital organs whenever diabetes is out of control. Take charge of your health, weight and quality of life by implementing the practical recommendations in this guide.

The good news is that diabetes, high cholesterol, blood pressure, heart disease, smoking, obesity and inactivity are controllable and respond to both treatment and lifestyle changes. However, left unchecked, these diseases will seriously impair your health and quality of life, and often, move you towards an untimely death.

Diabetes is like a sword with 20 sharp edges only controllable by *you*. Out of control, this sword can destroy you more quickly than you can imagine. The edges of this sword are sharp. Be safe by following the steps outlined here in this guide.

Since I started my pharmacy practice in 1987, I have observed thousands of people with chronic conditions suffering from preventable complications, which they most likely would not have had, had they been properly informed. Every day I witness diabetics with complications such as amputations, high blood pressure, high cholesterol, strokes, heart attacks, blindness, neuropathy, and heart disease and kidney failure.

The little time that doctors, nurses and pharmacists spend with people who suffer from chronic illnesses is shrinking. It is estimated that a doctor spends an average of "three or four minutes" with each patient. Prescription volume is increasing and the little time available to counsel patients, especially those with multiple chronic conditions, is shrinking even further.

The massive number of people who have preventable, chronic illnesses are falling through the cracks of our healthcare system and go on to succumb to complications since they are ill informed about their conditions. A large percentage of people who take prescriptions for preventable, chronic conditions can cut back on medications and prolong their lifespan *if* they make the right lifestyle choices and implement the changes necessary to achieve that goal.

As a pharmacist behind the pharmacy counter, I can reach a limited number of people. *My hope is that this guide can bring the message to the broader population and help prevent or even reverse diabetes and its complications.* **It is crucial that people claim responsibility for their health and make favorable lifestyle choices. If you act on the information provided here in this guide, you will be navigating toward safer shores and reaping the benefits of lifelong good health. It is simpler than you might imagine.**

No one but you can make the necessary choices. If you let this guide collect dust, disruption of your quality of life is imminent.

Introduction

My mission in having become a pharmacist and writing this guide is to help you live a healthier life. This guide is the compass that will point you in the direction of diabetes control. Take action now, and you will feel these benefits begin.

IMPORTANT MESSAGE

This guide was written for the patient, the regular person who visits a doctor's office, *avoiding high-ended literary terminology and technical phrasing* that is nearly indecipherable except by medical professionals.

The information that is provided in this guide is what you would get if you came to my window at the pharmacy—or rather, what I would like to tell you if only I had enough time. *This guide is deliberately written in a conversational style, addressing you, the reader, directly.* I am attempting to reach out to as many people as I can from the most educated to the least. I went to great lengths to simplify the terminology so that all readers can understand the information and act on it right away.

The messages in this guide are simple enough for anybody to understand, yet up to date and powerful enough to literally change your life. To bring your diabetes under control, to prevent deadly complications, to enjoy a normal lifespan and the best quality of life YOU, THE READER, NEED TO BE THE PRIMARY PARTICIPANT IN YOUR WELLBEING—AND YOU CAN DO IT! I urge you to read carefully and ACT on the information provided in this guide. You may need to reread some of the sections several times to master the information completely, but if you do, I believe in my heart you can get well.

Unfortunately, we pharmacists never seem to have enough time on our hands at the pharmacy. With this guide, I have tried my best to provide you with all the information you might need, presented in the simplest possible way to manage your disease successfully.

My main message is to let you know that favorable Lifestyle Changes are at the heart of keeping your condition at bay.

I relay this information to you from my perspective as a pharmacist with 20 years of experience. I want to help bridge the gap in health care I have witnessed during my practice.

This Guide is by no means an exhaustive volume. For instance, when I am counseling you about diabetes's various types, you will not find a list of ALL possible causes listed for each type, only the most common causes. The same applies for medication: you will not find a list of ALL possible side effects, drug interactions or every last detail about a medication, just the most up-to-date, practical information.

This guide is meant to be a complement to information you might get from your doctor, nurse practitioner, CDE provider, pharmacist, dietitian or other health care provider. I base my technical information and recommendations on the sources provided in "Sources of Data" at the end of this guide. For further details, contact your trusted health care professional, the American Diabetes Association at 1-800-342-2383, or log on to: www.diabetes.org and the other websites provided at the end of the guide.

Action Step 1:
Understanding Diabetes

HOW IS DIABETES AFFECTING AND IMPACTING OUR SOCIETY?

Diabetes is a mushrooming disease of epidemic proportions in the U.S.A. and worldwide. It is becoming one of the largest medical challenges of the 21st century. Pierre Lefebvre, President of the International Diabetes Federation, has been quoted saying: "As diabetes spreads across the globe, the world is heading for one of the biggest health catastrophes it has ever seen."

Diabetes affects over 125 million people worldwide, and more than 17 million in the United States. According to the American Diabetes Association, diabetes-related complications due to **UNCONTROLLED diabetes cause more than 200,000 deaths** in the U.S. annually, a staggering **75% of which are the result of debilitating strokes, heart and artery disease complications.** Up to a whopping **73% of adult diabetics have high blood pressure, which could lead to strokes, heart attacks and premature deaths** if not brought under control and it can be. **UNCONTROLLED diabetes is the cause of over 45% of new cases of kidney failure and up to 70% of nerve damage called Neuropathy** causing loss of sensation, pain and numbness in the hands and feet leading to amputations. **UNCONTROLLED diabetes is the cause of over 60% of ALL leg and foot amputations, and also is the LEADING cause of blindness in people between the ages of 20 to 75.**

These statistics are startling, they don't lie and they keep on climbing. This correlates with an all time rise in obesity and inactivity (solutions to the weight epidemic is discussed in details in action step 4). You have the power not to be part of these statistics. You can avoid these complications. You don't have to suffer a major blow to your quality of life and constantly live under the threat of being attacked by those vicious diabetes complications, which will slash years from your lifespan.

We now have evidence that you can prevent these complications. Revealing landmark trials such as the "UKPDS," "DCCT" and many others prove this finding. Keep your diabetes "under control" (see action step 3 to find out what and how to keep the various crucial parameters "under control") and live to tell stories to your grand and great grand children instead of having your children say "my father died from diabetes at age 52. He also was very heavy" or "my sister who is 48 lost both legs to diabetes and she is now in a wheel chair," or "my mom, now 56 years old, has been legally blind for several years and now her diabetes got so bad that she has to go the hospital for dialysis 3 times a week and be strapped to a machine for several hours each time to have her system cleansed. She is on a lot of medications."

You can bring diabetes under control. If you act on the simple tips provided to you in the 5 easy action steps of this guide, you can regain control of your weight, your health and your life and at the same time have natural lifespan complications free. Anyone can do it.

More alarming are the six million people in the U.S. who may have undiagnosed diabetes and have been harboring it for more than 10 years! These undiagnosed individuals, with blood sugar levels of 700 points (mg/dl) or more are walking hazards. These people must be identified and treated immediately. By getting a simple blood glucose test, you can determine if you are at-risk for diabetes.

The number of diabetes incidents is on the rise. The U.S. Center for Disease Control (CDC) reports that the number of Americans affected with diabetes has increased by an alarming 61% since 1991. It is estimated that 1 in 3 people born in the U.S. will develop diabetes. African-Americans, Hispanics, Asian Americans and Pacific Islanders are two to three times more likely than Caucasians to develop diabetes. **What is even more alarming is the all time sharp rise in the number of obese children diagnosed with Type 2 diabetes or likely to become diabetic.**

Obesity and the diabetes epidemic, in kids and adults alike, is fueled by poor lifestyle choices such as inactivity due to extensive hours of TV watching, sitting behind a computer or playing video games. Moreover, this dangerous epidemic is compounded when people couple inactivity with consuming "large portions" of typical "Western diet" foods such as pizza, hamburgers, hot dogs, French fries, fried food, salty chips, crackers, packaged and processed snacks, cookies, chocolate, ice cream, alcohol and, most importantly, sugar-loaded soft drinks. These foods are nutrient-deficient, very low in beneficial fiber, and very high in fats and sugars which largely and directly contribute to weight gain and promotion of chronic disease.

The blame for children's obesity and the diabetes epidemic within that age group goes to their parents and to school systems that allow kids to eat unbalanced portions of "junk food" and offer, on a daily basis, nutrient-deficient foods to these children and easy access to large amounts of soft drinks which alone is responsible for over 30% of obesity in USA. Parents and teachers also act as negative role models to kids if the parents and/or teachers are obese, if they smoke, or if they lead sedentary lifestyles.

Recent "CDC" data indicates that more than 58% of adults in the United States are overweight, and of those, 21% are obese, 60% do not engage in regular physical activity, and more than 25% of all Americans do not engage in *any* physical activity. The enormous rise in obesity is a clear link to the alarming rise in Type 2 diabetes. Since people with Type 2 diabetes account for about 90% of all diabetics, and since Type 2 diabetes is directly lifestyle-related, then a reverse trend will only be seen when people become more informed about diabetes and make favorable lifestyle changes.

There will NEVER be a MAGIC PILL, a panacea or a cure-all for obesity. The only way to control diabetes is to monitor the crucial parameters, take your medications daily as prescribed, and regain control of your weight by making favorable lifestyle choices and by managing stress. We will discuss each of these Action Steps in detail within this diabetes guide.

Your rewards will be avoiding premature death from complications due to diabetes, and enjoying the best quality of life.

What Is Diabetes?

Diabetes is the inability to transfer sugars in blood into the sugar-storage sites of your body, the muscles and liver. Sugars, called carbohydrates, are found mainly in cereals, rice, bread, pastas, potatoes, milk products, fruits, fruit juices and sweets. When we consume these foods, they pass from the stomach into the intestines and get broken down to the most basic sugar form, glucose.

Glucose (sugar) normally moves into the blood via a web of blood vessels that are connected to the intestines. When the movement of glucose into the blood stream raises its average level above 100 points (mg/dl), it triggers the secretion of a hormone called insulin from the pancreas. When insulin is secreted into the blood, it causes the excess glucose (sugar) to be stored in muscles and liver cells. It is stored in a form called glycogen, which may be used at a later time as an immediate source of energy.

This energy is used for activities of up to three minutes: lifting or throwing an object, running away from danger, sprinting, stop-and-go actions such as a short walk, or any sports activity. Some people have impairment in their insulin production or in the functioning of their insulin. This insulin impairment causes the level of glucose to rapidly rise above the 100-point mark, and that is the condition we call diabetes.

High sugar levels, left untreated, can gradually cause damage to vital tissues, such as blood vessels, the nervous system, kidneys, heart and arteries. This can cause debilitating strokes, heart disease, erectile dysfunction, loss of sensation or pain in the feet and hands, leading to leg amputations, kidney failure and blindness.

How Many Types of Diabetes Are There?

There are many types of diabetes:

Type 1 Diabetes

Type 1 Diabetes is when someone can produce little or no insulin, due mainly to immune and genetic (inherited) defects in the pancreas. People with Type 1 Diabetes create approximately only 10% of all of people diagnosed with diabetes. Type 1 can occur at a relatively young age, especially during childhood. At the time of diagnosis, people are usually of average weight, experiencing weight loss; frequent urination, blurred vision and dry mouth and their blood fasting sugar are way above 125 points (mg/dl). Type 1 diabetics have to depend on insulin use for the rest of their lives, in order to survive and making good lifestyle choices is integral to diabetes control. Oral Diabetes medications that are Sensitizers (see detailed discussion of this group of drugs in Action Step 2 right after the Insulin section) can be prescribed along with Insulin for people with Type 1 which can help reduce the amount of daily insulin used. Also leading and maintaining an active Lifestyle and making favorable food choices and raising your fiber intake can all help bring Diabetes under control and reduce the amount of total daily insulin dose (decisions about insulin dosing can ONLY be made by your doctor). Refer to Action Step 4 for a detailed discussion on how to start and maintain an active Lifestyle and make favorable food choices.

Impaired Glucose Tolerance or Pre-diabetes

This is a condition where glucose levels are higher than normal but not enough to be diagnosed as diabetes namely at a range from 100 to 125 mg/dl on a fasting state (first thing in the morning before eating). Typically, people in this category are overweight or obese. They are people who consume large amounts of "junk food" (nutrient-deficient food, loaded with sugars and unfavorable sources of fat such as animal fat, butter, margarine and Trans Fatty Acids that are found in the majority of packaged snacks) and have sedentary lifestyles; they also have high cholesterol and triglycerides and have low HDL (the good cholesterol). Studies show that these people will eventually develop diabetes and other preventable chronic ailments, such as: high cholesterol, high blood pressure and heart disease, "unless" they are identified early and the person starts making favorable lifestyle choices.

Gestational Diabetes

Gestational diabetes affects some women during pregnancy and is characterized by consistently higher than 95 points (mg/dl) on a fasting state first thing in the morning, and over 120 points 2 hours after a meal. Most women who suffer from Gestational Diabetes will return to having normal blood glucose levels after delivery. Up to 45% of women who develop diabetes during pregnancy may progress to having full-blown diabetes later in life unless they make favorable lifestyle choices and change their eating and activity habits. The *main predisposing factors* for gestational diabetes are family history of diabetes, obesity *and sedentary lifestyles*. It is crucial that women at risk be identified, since high blood sugar causes fetal harm.

Who Should Test?

All women, early on in their pregnancy, who have the following criteria must be tested for high blood sugar; women who are: overweight, over the age of 25, who have family history of diabetes, those who belong to ethnic groups other than Caucasian, those who have previously had gestational diabetes, or who have previously delivered large babies over 9 pounds.

Treatment

Gestational diabetes is initially treated with Lifestyle interventions such as making balanced food choices and increasing activity as described in Action Step 4. If fasting (first thing in the morning before eating) blood sugar is not brought to 95 points (mg/dl) or to 120 points 2 hours after lunch or dinner then Insulin is the ideal drug that is used. Your doctor will decide which insulin product and dose is appropriate for you. (See the discussion about insulin in Action Step 2).

Type 2 Diabetes

Type 2 diabetes, on the other hand, usually affects people later on in life, after the age of 25 or 30. However, Type 2 Diabetes has alarmingly been plaguing children at a much younger age than ever witnessed. Kids as young as 15 and 17 who are obese and leading sedentary lifestyles and commonly seen in grocery stores shopping while riding electric shopping scooters, are now diagnosed with Type 2 Diabetes. About 90% of people with diabetes have Type 2. People with Type 2 Diabetes produce insulin from their pancreas, but due to lifestyle factors such as *obesity and inactivity* the insulin is not able to perform and move the extra sugar from the blood into the muscle and liver cells, resulting in the buildup of sugar levels in the blood. This defect is referred to technically as insulin resistance. The diagnosis for Type 2 Diabetes is when people have a fasting (before eating in the morning) blood sugar level of 126 points (mg/dl) and over on 2 separate readings.

Type 2 Diabetes can be of hereditary origin. Non-Caucasians are more predisposed to getting it. But the vast majority of people get it due to inadequate lifestyles such obesity, overeating and sedentary lifestyles. A staggering 75% of people with diabetes are *obese and inactive*. This lends to the worsening of their conditions. I witness this trend every single day in my pharmacy practice. People drop off several prescriptions for diabetes, cholesterol and blood pressure, and they sit the entire time in the pharmacy waiting area. When I counsel them about their medications and suggest they might increase the amount of daily walking, their invariable answer is, "I don't have time." Sometimes, they drop off their prescriptions and go food shopping; they bring back a cart full of bacon, cookies and other packaged snacks such as popcorn, jugs of soft drinks, pretzels, butter, white bread, and let's not forget the cigarettes!

People with Type 2 Diabetes may be treated with: medications, either taken by mouth and/or through insulin injections, *and by making favorable lifestyle choices*. Medications alone without an active lifestyle will never be an efficient way to control diabetes and/or other chronic lifestyle-related diseases. Your doctor has many medication options from which to choose. What is important is to *get diabetes under control in order to avoid deadly complications!* **Your health is your responsibility, and staying in close contact with your doctor and pharmacist is the only way to avoid diabetes complications and hugely important in keeping your diabetes under control.**

The message that I bring you is that, "You are not doomed." Certainly, you can control diabetes, but **you have to be aware of some simple facts and act on them. Inaction will cause these deadly ailments to creep up on you and systematically destroy your internal organs and claim your life prematurely.** You can become involved, seriously and consistently, in your health; take the lead and the primary responsibility for managing your health and disease! It is simpler than you think.

If you take charge of this responsibility, you reap the benefits of living your lifespan to the fullest, enjoying the best quality of life. It is very simple. You just have to *take charge* by starting to apply the reliable, simple, and practical recommendations in this guide.

IDENTIFICATION OF THOSE WHO ARE DIABETIC BUT HAVE NOT YET BEEN DIAGNOSED AND THOSE WHO ARE PRE-DIABETIC

Proper and early identification IS A MUST. What you don't know can indeed hurt you. Early detection allows people to take action before there are serious consequences. Immediate weight reduction, even as little as 5 to 7 pounds, can help you regain sugar control, reduce your blood pressure and cholesterol. You *can* lose these 5 to 7 pounds by making favorable food and activity choices, as recommended in my Learning to Make Favorable Lifestyle Choices section (Action Step 4). These wise choices can bring the situation under control.

People who have any combination of the following criteria should test for blood sugar at least once a year during a yearly doctor check up:

• People who are overweight or obese • People who are sedentary • People with a family history of diabetes • Women with a history of gestational diabetes or who have given birth to babies over 9 pounds • People belonging to the following ethnic groups: African-Americans, Hispanics, Native Americans, Asian- Americans, Pacific Islanders	• People with high blood pressure • People with high cholesterol • People with heart disease • Smokers • People who have symptoms of continuous thirst, and who experience frequent urination, fatigue, sudden vision problems, or numbness and/or tingling in the hands and feet

If your blood fasting sugar is below 100 mg/dl then you are not diabetic. *If your fasting blood sugar level is between 100 and 125 mg/dl, then you are considered glucose intolerant and/or are suffering from a condition called pre-diabetes.* **This means that you are about to have full-blown diabetes unless you start making favorable lifestyle choices as recommended in Action Steps 4 and 5.** *If your fasting blood sugar, however, is 126 mg/dl and over on 2 separate readings then this* **is** *a diagnosis for diabetes.*

I'd like to share a story. Ever since I started pharmaceutical practice in 1987, I tried, whenever possible, to become more involved with my patients. I didn't want to just be a dispensing pharmacist. Through my constant communications with my patients, I realized that only a small minority were informed and took appropriate action to bring their condition under control. They lived happily since their decision to take that control. Unfortunately, the vast majority had the "I don't care," or the "it is not going to happen to me" and "my health is someone else's responsibility" type of attitude. They paid the ultimate price.

Diabetics who espoused the latter approach had the worst outcomes and eventually developed most of the diabetes complications previously listed. I was very impressed by the actions of some patients who I would counsel; some over 80 years old, had diabetes but were persistent in their action to keep their condition under control from the moment of their initial diagnosis. They looked and felt good and they enjoyed the ultimate quality of life. **It can be done. You can live a long and healthy life despite being a diabetic, IF you keep its complications in check** by becoming more informed and by being proactive and employing the information you receive from this guide. That's all it takes.

Through my work, I have also encountered young people with diabetes in their 20's, 30's, and 40's who either have been misinformed, are in denial, have given up or do not want to take their condition seriously. They are overweight, smoke, and are inactive. These people act the way they do because they do not want to "feel" different than others and because they think that they have to be deprived of some foods and sweets for the rest of their lives. **That's old thinking; it is no longer the case!** They are misinformed, and the good news is they can enjoy eating from all the food groups in a balanced fashion as will be discussed in "Action Step 4": Learning to Make Favorable Lifestyle Choices. Any diabetic can lead a very normal and very active life, just like non-diabetics and **without being deprived from any food**. This guide will provide you with the necessary tools to achieve just that.

Now that you understand a little better your Type of diabetes and realize that you can make a major difference to the better in your quality of life, a call to action was upon you yesterday. If you want to have the blessing of a normal and a natural lifespan, then **adopt and start implementing, NOW, the 5 Action Steps** of this guide. You have already completed the first step, which is grasping a better understanding of diabetes and becoming more informed about your condition. Now let us climb to the next Action Step.

WHAT YOU ABSOLUTELY MUST KNOW AT A GLANCE FROM ACTION STEP 1

1. Understand your type of Diabetes (starting Page 24).

2. It is absolutely crucial to check out the criteria table on Page 28 in order to have:
   - All those who have diabetes and don't know it be identified and treated immediately and start implementing lifestyle changes, as discussed in Action Step 4, to prevent deadly complications *and*
   - All those who are pre-diabetics but not yet have it be identified immediately and start taking preventive actions to avoid full-blown diabetes by starting to immediately employ lifestyle changes as recommended in Action Step 4.

Action Step 2:
Get to Know Your Diabetes Medications

During my pharmacy practice, I realized that most people have a stigma about taking medications for prolonged periods of time for their chronic conditions. Consequently, they might make personal and ill-informed treatment decisions such as stopping their medications, or taking them intermittently to save money, or running out of medications and not taking the time to renew it in a timely fashion, or for various other reasons they interrupt the flow of the treatment without consulting with their pharmacist or doctor. **This is a dangerous practice and can lead to dire consequences.**

Throughout the history of my practice, day in and day out, I heard the same following statements from patients who either stopped taking their medications or were not taking them appropriately:

- "I take my blood pressure medication only when I'm not feeling good, and I usually can tell when I need it!"
- "I stopped taking my medications because I felt better, and my diabetes is doing good."
- "I can't afford my diabetes medications or my cholesterol medications, so I only have been taking them 2 or 3 times a week."
- "I did not take the blood pressure medication that the doctor prescribed because I don't want to have to take it for the rest of my life."
- "I don't take my cholesterol medications because I don't want my body to get used to it, and I don't want that medication to take over my body."
- "I told my wife to stop taking her blood pressure medications because I don't want her to get addicted to them."
- "The side effects that I read about my blood pressure, my cholesterol and diabetes medications were awful, so I stopped taking them because I thought it was dangerous to my health."
- "My sugar levels were good and never higher than 160 first thing in the morning, so I decided to not take the diabetes medications any more."

- "I don't want to take blood pressure medication and cholesterol medications for life because there's nothing wrong with me!"
- "I have not been taking my diabetes, cholesterol, and blood pressure medication since I moved here about nine months ago. I'm still looking for a doctor in this area."
- "It has been days since I ran out of my diabetes medications and my doctor has not okayed the refill request you people in the pharmacy have placed with his office!!

By the way, whenever you are taking any kind of chronic medications and the pharmacy is calling the doctor for you to renew your prescription, always ask for a medication loaner if you are out. Sometimes pharmacy personnel forget to ask if you ran out of your medications, but never interrupt your treatment and always ask for a medication loaner, and any pharmacy will be glad to do so.

First off, let me dispel some myths and provide general guidance regarding the chronic medications intake for any chronic condition. *Never* make personal treatment decisions without consulting with your pharmacist or doctor. Please know that you should have no ill feelings AT ALL if you take medications for any conditions for any length of time. If you have pain or have an infection or a cold, your doctor prescribes medications to treat them. You probably take a multivitamin or a calcium pill daily and for life (if not, you should).

The absolute same situation applies to any other chronic condition, including diabetes, high cholesterol, high blood pressure, depression, sexual dysfunction, heart disease or any other condition. It has been shown by numerous trials that the drugs available to treat these conditions are truly lifesaving, as they keep your blood sugar, blood pressure, and cholesterol or the condition being treated at bay; and, consequently, all sorts of fatal complications are averted. **We truly should feel so lucky that we are living in this era of advanced medicine and medicinal technology.**

Do not be reluctant, not for a minute, to take your medications diligently, and don't make any changes without informing your pharmacist or doctor. Taking your medications intermittently or when you think you need them does not provide you with the protection from controllable deadly complications. Only when you take your medications daily, at regular intervals, as prescribed, will you get the best protection from the medication.

This does not mean that you should not question what you have been prescribed. You should be informed; if in doubt, you "should," question what your doctor has prescribed and you can call the pharmacist and ask questions, or you can secure a second opinion by an alternate doctor.

If you are concerned about side effects, which you read about in the leaflet that accompanies the medications, talk to your pharmacist about your concern before making any decision to stop the medication. Professionals can interpret these side effects or these concerns of yours in a different and clearer way than a non-professional can. Most of these side effects are minor and manageable and occur in a very small percentage of people.

When your doctor decides on a medication course, he or she, weighs the following: benefits vs. consequences; and the benefits of these drugs, most often, far outweighs any consequences. So *never* make personal decisions and uninformed decisions about any kind of medication without consulting with professionals first because if you do you could be putting yourself in harms way.

Also, It is very important **not** to share or "prescribe" your medication to anyone else. Likewise, do not accept your friend's, neighbor', uncle's, ant's, mom's or anyone else's medication and do not allow any one "prescribe" their medications to you. Only your doctor can diagnose and prescribe medications to you. Consult with your pharmacist for Over The Counter recommendations and about any other inquiry regarding any of your medications.

In this section about medications and in the next section about monitoring diabetes complications, you will find a simple description of the drugs you might be taking, along with what you should know and what you should do about problems, should they arise, and you should also be aware of side effects and drug interactions.

The purpose of the medication section of this guide is to give you general counseling on the medications you could be taking, some possible side effects or drug interactions as if you are getting counseling from your pharmacist at the pharmacy counseling window. This is not a complete list of all side effects and drug interactions available in the literature but the most common ones that *may* affect you. *Knowing and interpreting* the more extensive and technical information should only be the burden and responsibility of health professionals.

Any time you feel something is "not right," when it comes to taking any medication, or if your pills look different from what you have been taking, or if you have any other concern, contact your pharmacist or doctor and discuss that matter with them before taking any action. The medications you are taking for diabetes, blood pressure, cholesterol or any other purpose will not take over your body and will not be addictive. Each group of medications works in different ways to control the condition from which your body is suffering. Once you stop taking the medication, it slowly leaves your body, and so does its protective benefit.

In some cases, chronic diseases such as blood pressure, diabetes, high cholesterol and heart disease can be reversible if they were a result of poor lifestyle choices, such as obesity, inactivity and smoking; if these lifestyles are changed for the better, the weight is lost, and more favorable choices are made by each and every one of us. However, any decisions about stopping, starting your medications or changing your dosage should always be made by your doctor, not you. But even If you remain on medications for your chronic condition permanently, and most likely you will, then this is a good thing because those medications will save your life if taken as prescribed.

What matters here is that your goal should be to keep all your disease parameters under control in order to avoid complications and to experience the best quality of life. *There should be no stigma about taking medications anymore; think of them as the wonder vitamins that will literally save your life.* **Always remember that, whether your doctor decides to put you on medications or not, you must begin to or continue to make favorable lifestyle choices with regard to food and activity choices. Favorable lifestyle choices should always accompany drug intervention. These choices are at the very heart of averting disease complications.**

Before we start our discussion of the various medications that are available to treat diabetes, it is crucial to your safety to **become familiar with the signs of low blood sugar attacks**, which these drugs may cause. It is important to note that monitoring your blood sugar daily by owning and using a blood sugar monitor from the pharmacy, as will be discussed in Action Step 3, is paramount to detecting blood sugar dips below the recommended levels, and this monitoring is crucial in the prevention of these attacks. Once dips in blood sugars are detected, they can be rectified with the solution, which I will provide next.

Hypoglycemia

Critical Signs of Hypoglycemia (Or Low Blood Sugar Attack)

NOTE: "Any" of the following could be signs of low blood sugar. You do not have to experience all of these symptoms during a low blood sugar attack. You could be having a blood sugar attack with only one or two of these symptoms apparent. **People with Type 1 Diabetes may not be able to experience any of these symptoms and still be at a grave risk of low blood sugar attacks.** Consequently, it is vital for people with Type 1 to be diligent on monitoring their blood sugar several times daily before every insulin injection, 2 hours after lunch and before bedtime.

Signs of Low Blood Sugar:

- Nausea
- Dizziness
- Shakiness
- Sweating
- General ill feeling

Solution for Hypoglycemia (Or Low Blood Sugar)

Any time you are on insulin (or any medications you take by mouth for diabetes), you must have on-hand what are called Glucose tablets (available in many flavors) that you buy from any pharmacy store for about a dollar and a half per pack. *Keep those glucose tablets on you all the time.* Do not leave them at home or in the car, but keep them with you or close by. At the first sign of any of the symptoms mentioned above, **take one Glucose tablet out of the package and dissolve it in your mouth, and as soon as it dissolves, dissolve another 2 or 3. If you have access to a blood sugar monitor then try to take an immediate reading if possible. If your blood sugar is below 60 mg/dl then you need to dissolve up to 4 or 5 wafers back to back to bring it up to above a 100 mg/dl. If your blood sugar is 70 mg/dl then dissolving about 3 or 4 glucose wafers back-to-back is adequate.**

If low blood sugar is not treated immediately, it can progress to confusion, agitation, seizure, coma and or death in a very short period of time. This is a very serious matter that requires your attention. If glucose tablets are not available, then any kind of liquid sugar source will do: milk, fruit juice, and regular soft drinks (not diet soft drinks). Solid foods, chocolate or chocolate bars are **not** advisable because the fat or protein content delay the sugar absorption and **DO NOT** resolve this urgent situation. If loss of consciousness occurs from low blood sugar, EMS (Emergency Medical Services) needs to be called immediately; and, if available, using a Glucagon injection from an Emergency Glucagon Kit that you can purchase from any pharmacy with a prescription from your doctor, is the best remedy. So it is highly advisable that you keep a Glucagon Kit handy especially if you are on multiple insulin injections or a pump.

This section is for those who are curious. You may read this section at a later stage or read important information about those medications you are personally taking. If you wish to skip you can forward to Action Step 3.

The Various Classes of Medications Available To Treat Diabetes

Insulin

What Is Insulin and How Does It Work?

Naturally produced insulin from the body comes from what is called the "Beta Cells" in the pancreas when blood sugar levels from food consumed rise above 100 points (mg/ml). Insulin has 3 main functions in the body. First, when insulin responds to the rising blood sugar levels its main function is to usher the sugar to the muscles and liver and have it stored there thus reducing its presence in the blood. The next function insulin has is to help efficiently store the fat that we consume from food, in the fat deposits under our skin. Thirdly, insulin helps with the storage of the protein that we get from food into the muscle cells. The approach to treating diabetes differs and depends on the kind of diabetes that person has.

There are several categories of medications which people who have diabetes can take orally (by mouth) that will keep their condition and their diabetes parameters under control. And also, there is a drug called insulin that you inject under your skin; there is also the new insulin formulation that is inhaled by mouth and which has just become available for the treatment of Type 1 and Type 2 Diabetes. Generally, as a rule of thumb, when somebody is newly diagnosed with Type 2 Diabetes, oral medications are prescribed first.

Studies have shown that after approximately a decade on oral medications, many diabetics would require insulin treatment. This does not mean that their disease has worsened or that they're going "downhill." Several reasons some people with Type 2 Diabetes may eventually be put on insulin, first since people with this type of diabetes can have insulin production from their pancreas but due to their heavy weight coupled with inactivity their insulin cannot perform it's blood sugar lowering action which is referred to as insulin resistance. This leads to over production of insulin and thus over the years causing exhaustion to the pancreas' capacity to produce insulin.

Furthermore some oral diabetes medication belonging to the first group referred to as pancreas stimulators, which we will discuss right after the Insulin section, are highly effective in treating your diabetes and they work by stimulating your pancreas as well. Over the years these drugs coupled with your body's over stimulation of your pancreas' function can deplete insulin production. This is why it is of paramount importance to try to lose some weight permanently by learning how to make favorable food and activity choices as discussed in Action Step 4 since increasing activity and losing weight will make your body more sensitive and less resistant to insulin that is produced in your body. Consequently, as you start adopting a healthier lifestyle Insulin use may be delayed or avoided.

Insulin is a very effective way to treat diabetes and to reduce the sugar in your blood. The goal and aim of making favorable lifestyle choices is: when you become more active and make more balanced food choices (as recommended in the Action Step 4 of this guide) and you lose some weight, then your body will require less insulin to be produced; consequently, your dependence on medications can be reduced.

Insulin is, as I mentioned before, an effective way to treat diabetes. When it is time for you to use insulin, and when your doctor puts you on an insulin regimen, *it only means that a different and effective drug treats your diabetes.* Remember, regardless of the drug, and regardless of the agents used in treating your diabetes, **the most important factor is to keep your condition under control in order to prevent deadly complications.** Issues about your cholesterol and blood pressure and their treatment will be discussed in detail next in the Diabetes Complications section of this guide in Action Step 3. For now, let's start by discussing this wonderful drug called insulin.

Insulin works by causing sugar (glucose) that becomes available from the food we eat to be taken up by the muscles, the liver, and the fat cells. Also, insulin causes the fat from the food that we eat to be taken up by the fat tissue underneath our skin, and insulin will also cause the protein that we eat from food to be taken up by our muscles.

Side Effects

Some side effects of insulin usage include:

- Weight gain
- Worsening of insulin resistance
- Possible artery disease
- Hypoglycemia, (which is a low blood sugar attack. See section titled "Hypoglycemia" above for solutions)

Long-acting insulin such as Lantus, Humulin U and the most recent Levemir has the least potential to cause low blood sugar. All other insulin may have the potential to create this urgent and grave condition known as Hypoglycemia or low blood sugar.

Drug Interactions with Insulin

Some drugs may cause an increase in blood sugar when taken with insulin. Some of those drugs are:

- Diuretics such as HCTZ
- Drugs such as Prednisone
- Oral Contraceptives
- Beta Blockers such Atenolol, Metoprolol and Toprol

Solution

The solution for these drug interactions is to monitor blood sugar with a glucose meter several times daily as you regularly would and report to your doctor of any fluctuations so he or she can suggest a dose adjustment if any is needed.

Dosing of Insulin

Dosing of insulin is individualized and is determined only by your doctor (see Table 1 on the next page).

Table 1: Various Types of Insulin Available

Kind of Insulin	Name	Looks	Will Start Working Within	Will Last For	When to Use	Important Notes
Rapid Acting	Humalog (Lispro) Novalog (Aspart) Apidra (Glulisine)	Clear Clear Clear	Less than 50 min. Less than 25 min. Less than 45min.	3.5 h 3-4 h 3-4 h	15-20 min. before meals 15-20 min. before meals 15-20 min. before meals	
Short Acting	Humulin R (Regular) Novolin R (Regular)	Clear	Within 45 min.-1 h	3-6 h	30-45 min. before meals	
Intermediate Acting	Humulin N (NPH) Novolin N (NPH)	Cloudy	In 2-4 h	10-16 h	Inject morning and/or evening as prescribed by your doctor.	Roll gently in your hands before use
Long Acting	Lantus (Glargine)	Clear	In 4 h	24 h	Single injection/day, morning or evening	Long acting insulin causes the least hypoglycemia attacks (low blood sugar) if at all
	Humulin U (Ultralente)	Cloudy	In 6-8 h	18-20 h	Single injection/day morning or evening	
	Levemir (Detemir)	Clear	In 3-4 h	6-24 h	1 to 2 injections per day	

These insulin preparations are available in multiple use vials and are also available in a disposable PEN form or a reloaded cartridge form, for ease of locating and administering the dose prescribed by your doctor. The PEN form of injecting insulin eliminates the step of drawing insulin into a syringe.

Proper Injection Procedure and Mixing of Insulin

Most insulin can be mixed, with the exception of Lantus. When mixing a short acting insulin, such as Novolin or Humulin R, with an intermediate acting Novolin or Humulin N, always draw the clear "R" insulin first, and then draw the cloudy "N" into that same syringe. Here are the proper injection techniques:

1. Before starting any insulin injection, you must take a blood sugar reading. It is recommended that the blood sugar reading be taken before any meal; the blood sugar level should be below 110 mg/dl.

2. Wipe the rubber tip end of the insulin vial and the injection spot on your abdomen with an alcohol swab to make sure the areas where you draw blood and where the insulin will be injected are clean. Then let dry for a minute.

3. Roll the vial of the cloudy insulin "N" gently between your hands to warm the cold insulin and reduce discomfort after injecting it. Also, you roll gently and NOT vigorously to prevent bubble formation, which could affect the dose of insulin drawn and injected.

4. Draw air into the injection syringe equal to the total number of units prescribed of both kinds of insulin.

5. Inject air into the insulin vial via the rubber tip equal to the number of units of the "N" first; then inject the remainder of air into the "R."

6. As the syringe is still inside the "R," with one hand, flip the insulin bottle upside down and draw the number of units prescribed of the "R" with the other. Then insert the same syringe into the "N"; flip the vial in the same manner and draw the required number of units.

7. The abdominal area is the best site to inject insulin. Pinch the fat from the midsection of your abdominal area right above the navel; and with the other hand, inject the insulin straight into the fat. To avoid injecting insulin in the same spot and causing irritation to that site, rotate the injection sites and inject in different spots around that same area.

8. Dispose properly; all used needles and lancets from the glucose monitor, in specialized "Sharps" containers. Pharmacies normally carry or can order

these containers. If no sharps containers are available, dispose in tightly shut empty cans or empty juice bottles or small plastic bottles.

INSULIN STORAGE

1. Unopened insulin vials need to be stored in the refrigerator. Once you use insulin for the first time various kinds of insulin can be kept at room temperature as follows: Opened insulin vials can be kept at room temperature for up to 28 days and Levemir up to 6 weeks. Insulin pens must be kept at room temperature once you start using them. The Humulin 70/30 and Humalog 75/25 pens can remain at room temperature for 10 days; the NPH and Novolog mix pens for 14 days, the Humalog and Novolog pens for 28 days and the Levemir pen for up to 42 days. The Lantus' Opticlick digital display pen gets damaged at colder temperatures and can be kept at room temperature for up to 28 days.

2. Always check expiration dates.

PS: *Room temperature is around 77 F.*

Insulin Pump

Insulin pumps, in recent years, have become much smaller in size and very advanced in terms of the various functions they can perform. The pager-sized pump can be programmed by the user to deliver, continuously and automatically, the prescribed number of pre-meal and long-acting insulin units. Insulin is delivered from the pump into the skin via a tiny tube that is easily inserted by the user into the skin through a site insertion device.

Pumps are a very efficient way to deliver intensive insulin therapy, but they also require multi-task coordination and close monitoring of blood sugar up to 6 times or more per day; coordinate insulin amounts with meals consumed and carb-counting; be well-informed about the pump's proper operation, and be able to make quick adjustments to meals and activities if necessary; and make appropriate calculation adjustments to the proper insulin dose required for those changes. Generally, good pump candidates would have to be very well informed about all their disease aspects and be willing to remain in close contact with their doctor and pharmacist.

Malfunction of the pump unit can occur and can be problematic. The risk of hypoglycemia is inherently high and can cause serious problems if proper sugar monitoring is not implemented and meals are skipped. Pumps are expensive and some insurance programs can cover part of the pump's cost, which can average close to $5,000.00.

Exubera (Insulin—Inhaled by Mouth)

A long-awaited orally inhaled insulin has been approved to treat Type 1 and Type 2 Diabetes. In Type 2 Diabetes it can be used like other insulin products along with oral medications to treat Diabetes described above. This is the first kind of insulin, which can be inhaled through the mouth via an inhaler delivery system, instead of being injected under the skin. It is a rapid-acting form of insulin similar in speed of action to Humalog or Novolog and to be inhaled up to 3 times daily 10 minutes before meals. Using the inhaled Exubera insulin does not eliminate the need for injected insulin. Blood sugar needs to be monitored just like when insulin is being used.

How Does It Work and How Should You Use It?

The insulin powder is inside blister packets that can be activated by the inhaler device. Once the blister is activated the insulin powder is released as a cloud and fills a clear cylinder chamber connected to that handheld inhaler. The user should be standing or sitting upright. Immediately after its release, that insulin cloud has to be inhaled from a mouthpiece located at the top of that clear chamber. The user should breath out first away from the inhaler then seal that mouthpiece with his or her lips then inhale in one breath slowly and deeply all the way. Then the user should take the inhaler out of the mouth and hold his or breath for about 3 or 4 seconds then breathe out slowly. People with both Type 1 and Type 2 Diabetes can use Exubera.

Side Effects

Just like with other drugs for diabetes Exubera can cause low blood sugar (Hypoglycemia) which can be remedied as described in the insulin section (please review and be familiar with the signs and treatment of low blood sugar attacks in that insulin section above). Also after inhalation Exubera may cause a cough, dry mouth, throat irritation, chest discomfort and pain. Runny nose, slight trouble breathing and Sinus irritation may happen in about 3 or 4 % of people using Exubera. Lung function needs to be examined by your doctor at the start of the treatment with Exubera and periodically thereafter since this drug may lower lung function.

WHO SHOULD NOT USE EXUBERA?

- Smokers or those who have quit less than six months before starting Exubera
- People with any chronic lung diseases or compromised lung function including Asthma, chronic bronchitis, emphysema and lung cancer
- People under 18 years of age
- People who have Mannitol sensitivity

Let your Doctor know if you are pregnant, planning to be pregnant or breastfeeding since injected Human Insulin such as Humulin or Nonolin products are safer and preferred in these situations.

HOW IS IT AVAILABLE?

It is available in 1mg and 3mg blister packets. Each 1 mg packet is approximately equivalent to 3 units of injected "Humulin or Novolin R" insulin. One 3mg packet is equivalent to about 8 units of injected insulin. It is important to note that three 1mg blisters are NOT equivalent to one 3 mg blister. In the event that you run out of the 3mg blisters then two 1 mg blisters can be used momentarily until you are able to refill the 3mg ones at your earliest convenience.

Very Important General Tips about Insulin

- Insulin is a very effective way to treat Type 1 and Type 2 Diabetes. Getting on insulin is a good thing when it is required, and it does not mean your condition has taken a nosedive. In many people who have had Type 2 Diabetes for years and their oral diabetes medications have been used to maximum dosages and are not adequately controlling their blood sugar anymore, then using insulin products at this stage becomes necessary. Insulin, contrary to some peoples' beliefs, **does not** cause kidney failure, blindness or heart attacks; what causes all these complications is uncontrolled diabetes and blood sugar that has been allowed to go haywire by the diabetic who has not taken their condition seriously.

- **Never skip meals** when using insulin therapy or oral medication for diabetes treatment. If you have colds, have undergone a trauma, or don't have any appetite, try the liquid forms of nutrition that are specifically designed for people with diabetes, like Glucerna (yes, it has a well-balanced formula, and **the calories are needed). Don't get the sugar-free versions when you are replacing a meal,** *and* **keep up with taking the medications prescribed by the doctor.**

- When temporarily replacing meals with shakes, DO NOT GET THE SUGAR-FREE SHAKES, as you risk having an attack of Hypoglycemia (low blood sugar) after you use your insulin or oral medication. **Do not skip medications at any time, or make any changes to your dosage without consulting with your doctor or pharmacist. Increasing your daily activity level and eating three balanced meals and two fruit snacks daily from favorable sources as discussed in detail in the food section of Action Step 4, will help stabilize you sugar levels and prevent sugar ups and downs.**

- If you run out of your medications or your insulin because you don't have any more refills on your prescriptions, always ask your pharmacist or pharmacy personnel to loan you medications until they are able to get an okay from the doctor. Only Humalog requires a prescription. All other insulin can be bought without a prescription. However, if you use insurance, your pharmacy will require a prescription, even for insulin that does not require a prescription.

- Insulin can very effectively reduce A1C to the ideal level of 6 to below 7%, as is recommended by the American Diabetes Association (more on the A1C monitoring parameter in the monitoring section of Action Step 3).

Oral Medications to Treat Type 2 Diabetes

As discussed in the insulin section, insulin can be used for people who have Type 1 and Type 2 Diabetes. **Insulin can be used for people who have Type 2 diabetes when oral medications alone, after maximal doses of multiple drug combinations become less effective in bringing diabetes under control.** The medications taken by mouth only work in the presence of insulin that is being produced by your body. People who have Type 2 Diabetes still have insulin production, but that insulin is not used properly, and they need medications, such as the one that we will discuss in this section, to be taken by mouth to help that insulin work properly. There are several classes of oral diabetes medications that work in different ways and that can be combined together to help maximize the control of Type 2 Diabetes.

I. Long-Acting Pancreas Stimulators

Medications in this group stimulate the pancreas to secrete insulin. Specifically, these medications will stimulate what are called the Beta cells in the pancreas to increase insulin secretion. Drugs in this class include:

1. **Amaryl** (Glimeperide. Generic is available). Capacity to reduce A1C levels: 1.5 to 2% (A1C is a crucial parameter that measures average glucose levels over a period of 3 months. Ideally A1C level should be below 7%. Every 1% drop of the A1C level, closer to below 7%, will result in a 35% reduction in blindness and nerve damage (neuropathy). We will discuss this parameter in detail in the monitoring section.

2. **Glucotrol** or **Glucotrol XL** (Glipizide. Generic is available): Capacity to reduce A1C levels: 0.6 to 1%.

3. **Glyburide** (This a generic form): Starting dose: Capacity to reduce A1C levels: 0.6 to 1%.

<u>Possible Side Effects:</u> Low blood sugar (at the first sign of low blood sugar, dissolve 2 to 3 glucose wafers back to back in your mouth as discussed in the insulin section. See symptoms and solution of low blood sugar mentioned in the insulin section). Other side effects are weight gain, skin rash, dizziness, nausea and stomach upset.

What Should You Remember About this Class of Medications?

- Take with food.
- Do not skip meals.
- Watch for signs of Hypoglycemia (low blood sugar). Check blood sugar frequently, at least one to two times per day. These medications can cause a drop in blood sugar below normal levels; so keep glucose tablets handy to remedy this situation as discussed in the "Hypoglycemia" section above.

II. Short-Acting Pancreas Stimulators
How This Group of Medications Works

Medications belonging to this group work in a similar way as in Group 1, by stimulating the pancreas cells, however, in a slightly different and smarter way. This group of medications will stimulate insulin release from the pancreas, depending on the amount of glucose that is available in your blood. In other words, as the glucose levels come closer to the normal levels in the blood, the effect of these medications will start to dwindle.

Consequently, they place less demand and less pressure on the pancreas to secrete insulin. Medications belonging to this group are:

1. **Starlix** (Nateglinide. No generics available yet). Take with meals. Capacity to reduce A1C levels: 0.5 to 1%.

2. **Prandin** (Repaglinide. No generics available yet). Take with meals. Capacity to reduce A1C levels: Like Starlix.

Possible Side Effects: medications in this class have a low risk of low blood sugar. Other transient side effects can include flu like symptoms (fatigue and fever), body aches, dizziness, and possible stomach discomfort.

III. Liver Sensitizers
How This Group of Medications Works

The medications in this class sensitize the liver to decrease sugar production. Also the medications in this class cause the stimulation of muscle cells to take in the sugar from the blood and store it inside. This class of medications can only work in the presence of insulin that is still being secreted from the pancreas.

Medication name: **Glucophage** (Metformin, generic form available). Starting dose: 500 milligrams once a day for a week then gradually increase by 500 milligrams per week to a total of 1000 milligrams twice a day to minimize stomach problems. Maximum effective dose: 1000 milligrams twice a day. Take with meals. Capacity to reduce A1C: 1.5 to 2% (one of the most powerful drugs to reduce A1C).

Possible Side Effects:
- Stomach discomfort (the dose is gradually increased to reduce the incidence of stomach problems)
- Diarrhea
- Nausea and possible vomiting
- Anorexia or loss of appetite
- Metallic taste in the mouth.

Most of these side effects will subside after continued use of perhaps a week or two.

What You Should Know about This Medication:
- Metformin is a cornerstone treatment in Type 2 Diabetes. It can be used as a single first line treatment or in combination with drugs from other classes.

- This medication is **ideal for people who are overweight or who are obese.**
- There is definite evidence that Glucophage improves mortality in people with diabetes.
- Glucophage can be prescribed for people not yet diabetic but predisposed to become diabetic along with Lifestyle changes.
- **It causes weight loss**, which is a major advantage and a unique property of this drug. All others may actually cause a slight weight gain.
- It reduces triglycerides by 16%.
- It reduces LDL (bad cholesterol) by 8%.
- It raises HDL (good cholesterol) by about 2 or 3%.
- Insulin must be present, and the pancreas must be able to produce insulin for this medication to work.
- This is the most aggressive reducer of A1C levels.
- People who have kidney problems or congestive heart failure need to avoid taking this medication, as it may cause a serious condition called lactic acidosis.

IV. MUSCLE AND FAT SENSITIZERS

Medications belonging to this class sensitize the muscles and fat cells in the presence of insulin that is produced from the pancreas or that is injected to take the sugar from the blood stream and store it inside the muscle and fat cells. In a minor extent, they may also sensitize the liver to stop producing sugar. Medications belonging to this class are:

1. **Actos** (Pioglitazone): Capacity to reduce A1C levels: 1%. Take with breakfast.

2. **Avandia** (Rosiglitazone. No generic available yet). Take with breakfast. Capacity to reduce A1C levels: 1%.

<u>Possible Side Effects:</u>
- Weight gain.
- People who have more response to these medications may have the most weight gain.
- When this class of medication is combined with pancreas stimulators that belong to group 1 and 2 discussed above, this may cause further weight gain.
- Water retention which causes leg swelling.
- May worsen a pre-existing heart condition called congestive heart failure.

What You Should Know about This Class of Medication:

- This is a very important class of medications that is also integral to Type 2 Diabetes treatment. Weight gain can be manageable by favorable lifestyle choices. The benefits of these medications far outweighs any side effect.
- New studies are emerging, especially on Actos, for its heart protective properties, reducing complications of the heart besides reducing the blood sugar property.
- The Pancreas must be able to produce insulin for these drugs to work, just as with Glucophage.
- You will need to monitor your weight periodically (once a week).
- Medications in this class are almost always used in combination with other medications belonging to different classes.
- Your doctor will monitor your liver functions periodically.
- It takes approximately 8 to 12 weeks for maximum effects to start showing.

V. Sugar Absorption Blockers

Medications belonging to this class of drugs prevent the breakdown of sugar in the small intestine after a meal, and consequently delay the sugar being dumped into the blood. Medications belonging to this class:

1. **Precose** (Acarbose. No generic available yet). Take with meals. Capacity to reduce A1C: 0.3 to 1%.
2. **Glyset** (Miglitol. No generic available yet). Take with meals. Capacity to reduce A1C levels: 0.3 to 1%.

<u>Possible Side Effects:</u>

- Stomach upset and flatulence.
- Possible liver complications can happen. (Monitor liver function periodically every 3 months.)

What You Should Know about This Class of Medications

- Medications in this class can be used as single agents or in combination with drugs belonging to different classes.
- These medications can be effective in reducing the sugar absorption after a meal.
- Dose should be raised gradually to avoid stomach side effects and discomfort.
- Effect on keeping the blood sugar under control is modest.

- The effect of these medications depends only on the amount of sugar that is absorbed in a meal. If no sugar is consumed, they will have no effect.
- Take these medications with the first bite of food that contains any kind of carbohydrate or sugar.

VI. Januvia (Sitagliptin)

This is the first drug of a new class of oral diabetes medications that has just become available to treat Type 2 Diabetes only. It belongs to a class technically known as DPP-4 inhibitors which works to lower your blood sugar by increasing the amount of insulin produced by your body and decreases sugar production by your liver. This drug is prescribed alone or in combination with Glucophage, Avandia or Actos to treat Type 2 Diabetes.

Possible Side Effects: Common side effects are upper respiratory infections, runny nose, nasal congestion, headache, stomach discomfort and diarrhea.

What You Should Know about Januvia:
- It is an innovative and effective way to treat and bring diabetes under control.
- *It is prescribed in conjunction to balanced food and activity choices.*
- It is less likely to cause low blood sugar attacks.
- It is NOT indicated for Type 1 Diabetes.
- It is conveniently prescribed once daily.
- It is indicated for people over 18 years of age.
- You must inform your doctor if you have any kidney problems since dosage adjustment is necessary in this situation.
- It has not been studied in women who are pregnant and consequently should be avoided by pregnant women.

Possible Drug Interactions with Oral Diabetes Medications
(This not an exhaustive list of all drug interactions but the most common)

The following common medications will interact with possibly many diabetes medications raising or decreasing the effectiveness of these diabetes medications. Consequently your blood sugar may fluctuate up or down. When consuming any of the following medications, monitor your sugar frequently at least once or twice a day or more if you are on insulin, to see how the levels of sugar are being affected. Ideally, your sugar level before a meal should be below 110 mg/dl and above 70 mg/dl. Two hours after any meal it should be below 145mg/dl. If your blood sugar level has been stable and close to these numbers and then at the start of any of the following medications your sugar starts fluctuating then contact your doctor for a solution on dosage adjustment of any of the medications or your doctor may switch you to another one. Drugs that may interact with your diabetes medications are:

- Tagament (Cimetidine). This is an over-the-counter stomach-acid reducer. Preferably, use Pepcid, Zantac or Prilosec; these won't cause this drug interaction with diabetes medications.
- Tegretol
- Dilantin
- Some antibiotics: Cipro, Levaquin and Ketek
- Allopurinol

Several of the medications we have discussed are available in combinations in a single pill form. (See list below). The reason for this is to help people remember to take their medications when you take fewer medications less frequently, you will have a tendency to remember taking them and, consequently, keep your sugar under control. Some of those combinations are:

- Avandamet: a combination of Avandia and Glucophage (generic form is available)
- Glucovance: a combination of Glucophage and Glyburide (generic form is available)
- Avandaryl: a combination of Avandia and Amaryl (new release, no generic available)
- Actoplus Met: a combination of Actos and Metformin (new release, no generic available)
- Duetact a combination Actos and Amaryl (the most recent release, no generic available)

Recent and Innovative Drugs in 2006

Advancement in treating diabetes is at an all-time high. New agents belonging to new classes of medications, new ways of treating diabetes, and new methods of administering those drugs are emerging all the time. Three very potential drugs have already entered the market in 2006; they are Byetta, Symlin and the long-awaited inhaled insulin, **EXUBERA (see details in the Insulin section above).**

BYETTA (NEW DRUG—NO GENERIC AVAILABLE YET)

Byetta belongs to a new class of medications recently made available and is used to treat only Type 2 Diabetes; it is administered by injection under the skin, like insulin. It is not indicated to treat Type 1 Diabetes.

How Does It Work?

The way Byetta works is by improving the pancreas' function; it allows the pancreas to self-regulate the glucose levels within the body by assisting insulin in lowering blood sugar on a fasting state and after meals. Byetta is prescribed only in combination with drugs in section I as discussed earlier, such as Amaryl, Glucotrol, Glyburide, and also Metformin.

Starting Dose

The starting dose is 5 micrograms for the first month, injected under the skin twice a day (morning and evening 30 to 45 minutes before meals). Maximum effective dose: after 1 month, if the sugar control in the body is not adequate, then the dose can be increased to injecting 10 micrograms under the skin twice a day, morning and night. Impact on reducing A1C levels: Byetta, when administered with the oral diabetes medications mentioned above helps people with Type 2 diabetes achieve their A1C goal of below 7%.

Side Effects:

- Byetta can cause low blood sugar, especially when consumed with drugs such as Amaryl, Glucotrol, and Glyburide. (Glucose tablets should be with the user all the time and must follow instructions discussed in the "Hypoglycemia" section above on how to remedy this situation.)
- Nausea
- Dizziness
- Headaches
- Stomach trouble: vomiting, diarrhea, and stomach discomfort
- Feeling of agitation

Storage

Keep used and unused Byetta packages in the refrigerator. If you are traveling and do not have access to cool travel packs then it can be kept outside the fridge at about 77 degrees for up to 6 days and still remain stable. But ideally keep Byetta in the refrigerator. Ask the manufacturer for cool travel packs. If traveling longer than 3 or 4 hours then place Byetta in a plastic bag and keep insulated from direct contact with ice, freezer packs and moisture.

What Else You Must Know about Byetta:

- **People who have kidney problems or kidney failure must not use Byetta.** The same applies for people who have any kind of stomach or intestinal ailments.
- Byetta is only indicated for people who have Type 2 Diabetes. People who have Type 1 Diabetes must not use Byetta.
- Byetta can improve A1C levels.
- Byetta can cause **weight loss.**

Symlin (New Drug—No Generic Available Yet)

Likewise, Symlin is an innovative way to treat Type 1 and Type 2 Diabetes via injections under the skin. Symlin resembles a substance secreted along with insulin from the pancreas to help reduce blood sugar after a meal. When someone has diabetes, Symlin (when given along with insulin) works by reducing the speed at which the food in the stomach is broken down and transferred to the colon. This helps to reduce blood sugar peaks. Also it improves the appetite response and causes the user to eat less. Symlin causes a mild weight loss of 2 to 3 pounds initially.

Symlin is to be used only after other treatments have failed. Symlin is used along with insulin with or without oral medications. Symlin is to be injected under the skin before meals. Its capacity to reduce A1C is between 0.39% to 0.62% and studies have shown that Symlin, along with insulin, has helped its users ultimately to reach the desired A1C level of below 7%.

Side Effects:

- Hypoglycemia (low blood sugar attack). Refer to the insulin section for signs and treatment of low blood sugar attacks (hypoglycemia). As with other diabetes medications blood sugar need to be monitored several times daily.
- Nausea and vomiting is more prevalent at the start of the treatment and then decreases and subsides after a couple weeks. These side effects may be reduced if the Symlin dose is increased slowly and gradually to the required dose as instructed by your doctor.

Storage

After first use, Symlin can be kept either in the refrigerator or at room temperature for up to 28 days. An opened vial needs to be discarded after 28 days.

New Diabetes Drugs on the Near Horizon

RIMONABANT (NOT YET AVAILABLE ON THE MARKET)

This new drug, with its unique ability to treat several conditions at one time, will soon be available. Rimonabant is the first of a new class of drugs, which helps treat obesity, diabetes, high cholesterol and tobacco dependence, all at once. There is a receptor system in the brain referred to as the E.C. system, which is responsible for regulating hunger, nicotine dependence, and in part, insulin resistance. When people overeat or become overweight, or use nicotine or tobacco, they over-stimulate the E.C. system, and it becomes imbalanced. The drug Rimonabant helps bring balance to the system.

People who took 5 to 20 milligrams of Rimonabant per day were able to lose weight, and their diabetes became controlled, with A1C levels brought to desired levels. Those who smoked had much greater success quitting, their cholesterol profiles and insulin sensitivity also improved. Those testing this drug were also put on lifestyle modification, eating balanced diets and increasing their activity. The drug alone will not help all of these problems, but making more favorable lifestyle choices will be integral in advancing improvements. This drug is very promising, but lifestyle modification will always remain a crucial factor in improving people's health, preventing disease or complications, and improving quality of life.

It is normal practice for your doctor to put you on one or more medications for diabetes that belong to the various classes mentioned above. Only your doctor will make that choice of drugs or combination of drugs, assessing the dosages and frequencies that are right for you. I STRONGLY URGE YOU NOT TO MAKE PERSONAL DECISIONS REGARDING YOUR MEDICATIONS WITHOUT CONSULTING YOUR DOCTOR OR PHARMACIST FOR YOUR OWN SAFETY AND WELLBEING.

The Importance of Taking Aspirin Or Other Blood-thinning Medications

If you have diabetes, heart disease, or high cholesterol and you are not taking aspirin, you should. Thinning your blood helps prevent blood clots, a factor in major cardiovascular events such as heart attacks and strokes. If you have any of these ailments, especially diabetes, consult with your doctor before starting on aspirin, but every diabetic needs to be on a dose of enteric-coated aspirin ranging from 81 milligrams (Baby Aspirin) to approximately 325 milligrams. Studies have shown that benefits of thinning blood with 81 milligrams of aspirin are very similar to taking higher dosages about 160 to 325 milligrams. The difference is, people taking higher dosages may have more stomach side effects.

If you've already had a stroke or a heart attack, your doctor may elect to put you on a different blood-thinning medication such as Plavix or Coumadin, Trental, Persantine or Aggrenox. As we age and become sedentary, our blood naturally thickens. Remaining active as we grow older is a major contributor to thinning your blood, preventing heart complications, and offering an array of other benefits. Ask your doctor before starting on any blood-thinning medications.

Ask for Generic Drugs (They Are Just as Good and a Lot Cheaper); How to Bargain for the Best Medication Prices And Tips on Finding Cheaper Drugs

Throughout my practice, I've seen a common heart-breaking problem, people not taking medications because they are too expensive and they can't afford it. Doctors may prescribe expensive medications for diabetes, blood pressure or cholesterol, not realizing how much they cost or that your insurance may not cover them. I've had people, especially older folks, cry at my pharmacy counter, not able to afford the cost of their drugs. I was always able to find solutions and get them their drugs. In every medication category, there are drugs that are available in cheaper generics with the same quality as the brand names.

The FDA monitors generic drugs for quality, and all generics labs have the same quality-control regulations as the brand names. Ask your doctor to prescribe a drug that is available in generic form that your insurance covers or if you cannot afford the brand names. THE CRUCIAL FACTOR IS FOR YOU TO NOT INTERRUPT TREATMENT FOR THESE AILMENTS, OR YOU WILL BE IN HARM'S WAY.

Call the pharmacy chains and independents in your area and find out which of them will match other pharmacies' prices. Make a list of the drugs that you need, and call the pharmacies in that area to get a quote on medications. Then go to a pharmacy that will match prices and let them know the lowest quote you received for each medicine; ask them if they can match or beat that price.

You can buy a few days' worth at a time, but make sure to ask for their minimum charge per medication sale. Every pharmacy has a minimum set charge for every drug sale that can vary from $4.99 to $10.99 regardless of how few pills you buy. That means if the minimum charge is $6.99 for each medication sale, and you buy 10 pills costing only $3.99, their computer will default to charge you that $6.99 minimum.

Find out that minimum charge, and order enough medication so that minimum gives you the most medicine for your money. When you are dealing with one pharmacy (you should try to get your prescriptions in one pharmacy that you are most comfortable with unless you are traveling, because the personnel will get to know you and have all your medication records and can detect problems and drug interactions better than if you are a "pharmacy-hopper"). Also you get to know the pharmacy personnel and can wheel and deal better with familiar personnel. Generally, independent pharmacies, Wal-Mart, Sam's Club, and Costco have the cheapest prices but you need to call around and do your homework as other pharmacy chains can be competitive as well.

WHICH PHARMACY SHOULD YOU CHOOSE?

I suggest you select a pharmacy that is most conveniently located to your place of residence and one that you are most comfortable communicating with their pharmacists and technicians on duty. Cordial, caring and knowledgeable pharmacy personnel should be key criteria to selecting and establishing a good relationship with people at your local area pharmacy. Should any question regarding your medications come up, you should not hesitate to call your local pharmacist and feel comfortable talking to him or her. Pharmacists are very knowledgeable professionals who look out for your well-being. They are key in helping you manage your condition more efficiently and get you informed about your prescription and over the counter medications, possible side effects and warn you of potential drug interactions.

If you do not have insurance for your prescription medications then I would also select a pharmacy that offers competitive prices or willing to match or beat competitors. If you do have insurance then your co-pay on medications should be same regardless of what pharmacy you choose (check with your insurance regarding this and all other insurance related issues for clarification.) Consequently, customer service and patient care would be the main criteria for your pharmacy of choice. The advantage of pharmacy chains is that they are spread out throughout many parts of the nation and many have centralized records. Consequently, if you are moving to various locations then chances are that they can pull your record from any location. They are also keen on providing good customer service, convenient locations and the convenience of a wide variety of store merchandize and food products all in one location. Pharmacy chains carry throughout their stores extensive lines of Brand and Private Label competitively priced merchandize in a wide variety of product lines.

The advantage with independent pharmacies is a personalized service that you get with your neighborhood independent pharmacy as they get to know you by name and the medications you are on. Moreover, since independent pharmacies know that they have to compete with the giants in the business to stay afloat, they may offer extensive lines of products that pharmacy chains may not carry. It is not uncommon to find extended lines of medical supplies such as canes, bath tub chairs, extension commode seats, walkers, nebulizers, and many other supply lines; fertility drugs; injectable prescription medications and oddball prescription items that pharmacy chains usually don't care to stock in addition to the usual extended line of prescription drugs and over the counter brand and some

Private Label medications. They also offer competitive prices and bill most insurance plans just like the retail chains. Don't forget that fountain pharmacies still do exist and offer sumptuous meals and unique merchandise. Frequently, pharmacists operating in retail chains have been referring patients to local independent pharmacies for items they don't stock. Independent pharmacies including the Medicine Shoppe franchise, which is independently owned, are the bread and butter pharmacy operations of your local neighborhood.

> **WHAT YOU ABSOLUTELY MUST KNOW AT A GLANCE FROM ACTION STEP 2**
>
> 1. Get familiar with the types of diabetes medications you are using and take them EVERY DAY as prescribed and NEVER MAKE ANY TREATMENT DECISIONS TO STOP YOUR MEDICATION/S, OR TO CHANGE HOW OFTEN YOU TAKE THEM OR TO CHANGE THE DOSAGE WITHOUT CONSULTING WITH YOUR DOCTOR OR PHARMACIST (starting Page 36).
>
> 2. Get familiar with the signs of low blood sugar attacks (hypoglycemia) and the solution for it in the section titled "Hypoglycemia." Low blood sugar attacks are potentially serious and fast occurring and can be life threatening, unless you know what the signs are and how you can resolve the situation (Page 35).
>
> 3. **All people who have diabetes should be on blood-thinning treatment such as aspirin** or the other blood thinning medications that are available in order to avoid heart attacks or strokes. If you are not taking any blood-thinners then have your doctor recommend one for you (Page 54).
>
> 4. How to find real medication bargains (Page 54).

Action Step 3:
The Vital Importance of Monitoring Your Sugar, Cholesterol, Blood Pressure and Feet; Treatment of Cholesterol and Blood Pressure; What Complications Can You Prevent?

DIABETES COMPLICATIONS

Potential, Debilitating and Life-Threatening Complications of Diabetes

Diabetes is considered out of control if blood sugar readings are erratic, swinging between 150 one day and 400 the next. This can result from being overweight, smoking, uncontrolled eating (like there is no tomorrow), and being totally inactive (sitting at work every day and watching TV the rest of the week). I urge you to rethink your attitude if you tell yourself, "I don't care, nothing is going to happen to me" or "No matter what I do, it is not going to change a thing."

YOU CAN BE IN CONTROL OF YOUR DIABETES. You can bring your blood sugar under control and, contrary to what you might think, you still can have your favorite foods and desserts but in moderation and in balance. *Your* efforts are required to make this happen.

If your morning-fasting-sugar-readings keep climbing above 110 or 115, this excess sugar starts gradually and systematically causing disease and compromised function to your vital internal organs, such as your arteries, your heart, your kidneys, as well as your nervous system and can even result in Neuropathy causing blindness, sexual dysfunction, loss of sensation in your limbs, as well as tingling and pain in your toes, feet, and legs leading to amputation. Disease of the main arteries can lead to high blood pressure, high cholesterol, heart attacks and strokes. Kidney failure requires

dialysis and possibly a transplant, as well as death at a young age. Also high blood sugar makes you prone to severe infections and much longer healing time even with the use of antibiotics and women have a much higher incidence and more occurrence frequency of urinary tract infections and bacterial or fungal vaginal infections. These events can occur at any age.

Can you imagine going through the rest of your life in a wheelchair, without your legs, or without the ability to see, or while having pain in your feet or arms every minute of every day, or having a weak heart, or living without your kidneys at the age of 48, 55 or 63, while you can prevent and avoid all of this. Have you had enough bad news yet?

You can prevent all of this from happening by keeping your sugar, cholesterol, and blood pressure "under control" (as discussed further down in this action step 3), by taking your medications as prescribed (see action step 2), by making favorable food and activity choices (see action step 4) by reducing and managing your stress (see action step 5).

Take no action, and pay the ultimate price, dragging you through life as a result of totally preventable diabetes complications.

The Harsh New Reality for Cedrik, Who Did Not Take His Condition Seriously

I cannot get over what I saw one day at the pharmacy. Cedrik, a young man in a wheelchair, was trying to reach for an item from the over-the-counter section in front of the pharmacy where I was working one day. I rushed out to help him and offered my services. To my surprise, I saw a man in the prime of his life who could not have been more than 47 or 48, with both legs amputated from slightly above the knee all the way down. He was in front of the diet aid section trying to select a product to help him lose weight, since he was obese. So I started inquiring further, in order to have a better understanding of what his needs were.

When I asked him whether the amputations were due to an accident or disease, he replied with a regretful tone, that it was due to complications of diabetes; an answer somehow I was expecting. Then he went on to tell me that the reason he is in this mess is because he was not compliant with taking his medications regularly, he did not monitor his sugar levels daily. He only had his sugar levels monitored at the doctor's office with every visit once every 4 to 5 months. He also made very poor food choices, as he ate sweets and cookies as if there were no tomorrow. He also led, largely, a sedentary life, as he watched TV 5 to 6 hours a day; and at work, he sat behind a behind a computer ALL day long.

Most of all, he felt that he was not properly informed about his condition and did not know that he actually could have prevented these debilitating diabetic complications with which he was now afflicted. He got bits and pieces from various sources, and when he was due for a doctor's visit, his doctor would examine him then writes some prescriptions and would tell him that he would need to "lose weight" and "exercise" without going into details on how to do that. Doctors are very busy, overworked and do not have the luxury to spend 30 to 45 minutes with every patient and explain what foods to eat or what type of exercise to do. Doctors usually refer patients to dieticians to take care of that part. Likewise at the pharmacy the prescription volume keeps on increasing and the technician support allocated to help the pharmacists is usually not enough. Consequently, the pharmacists have less and less time to counsel patients.

He proceeded to tell me that had he taken his condition seriously he would be walking today and would not have lost his legs, and be confined to a wheelchair today. He, his wife, and their two beautiful daughters, had to pull together, having to make major adjustments; they have gone through very tough times, coming to terms with this new reality. He told me, if it were not for the support and love of his family, he would have given up a long time ago. I could not help but to empathize and feel his deep regret.

After this introduction to him, I began counseling him about the medications he was taking and about the importance of daily blood sugar and blood pressure monitoring; I urged him to report to his doctor any consistent fasting-sugar-levels above 110, and blood pressure levels above 130/80. I also pointed out that his doctor should have many medication choices to bring any and all uncontrolled readings down to the norm. I also indicated that his doctor would need to monitor his cholesterol and A1C levels periodically, every 3 months.

We also discussed weight loss issues, those that did not involve using any diet pills, but did involve making favorable lifestyle changes. I gave him tips on making food choices, focusing on foods high in fiber and low in sugar, and I urged him to have 3 balanced meals a day and two fruit snacks per day in between meals; I also advised him on portion control to help his sugar levels stabilize.

Since he suffered from a handicap that debilitated his legs, I customized my advice regarding activity accordingly. Since he was/is bound by a wheelchair, he needed/needs to depend on arm movements to generate health and heart benefits and to prevent further disease complications. I suggested he push himself on the wheelchair, in open space for 10-15 minute bouts, a couple of times a day. Also, I indicated to him, that if he had/has access to a gym, he could use some of the machines there that are designed for upper body movement, such as hand cycling and some rowing exercises which involve most of the upper body muscles and can be operated by hand movements. He could access these machines straight from his wheelchair. We also discussed him using some multilevel resistance rubber tubing, cheaply available at Wal-Mart, to work his upper body muscles 2-3 times a week.

Finally, I truly tried to assuage some of his discomfort by genuinely caring for him and by reassuring him that he was able to prevent further complications and damage "if" he took action immediately and kept all his disease parameters under control. He then shook hands with me and thanked me for the great advice I had given him, and he wished that other diabetics would learn from his lesson and become more actively involved in their health, in order to turn away all preventable complications.

Unfortunately, Cedrik's story is mirrored by millions of diabetics every day. My main concern during pharmacy practice is to help people who suffer from chronic conditions take more favorable actions, keep up with the various parameters that would keep their illness at bay, and report to their doctor anything that is out of control, reminding them to take their medications as prescribed and to continue making better lifestyle choices, and most importantly, prevent themselves from ending up like Cedrik.

Monitoring

Imagine You Are the Captain of a Boat
In the Atlantic Ocean without Navigation Gear

If you have diabetes and want to truly avert its deadly complications **WITHOUT** monitoring the various crucial factors along the way, you will most certainly be doomed.

Just picture yourself a captain on a boat who is stripped of all navigation tools in the middle of the Atlantic Ocean, where you are the only one on board, and you are attempting to reach the shore safely. Would you steer to the north or to the south? But where is north or south? Would you steer right or left; either way, you could be headed in the wrong direction and away from safety, all the while, you thinking you are headed in the right direction. You will never reach safety without the proper gear. The same applies to monitoring your blood sugar and blood pressure daily.

Once you know what your target is, regarding your blood pressure, cholesterol and sugar and where they need to be, then when you monitor daily, you will be able to tell whether you are on target or not. When levels go off target, then you can inform your doctor and take other lifestyle actions in order to regain control. Just like the captain of that boat, you have your navigation gear set on a target in the direction of the shore, and during the journey, you constantly take readings to see if you "are" still on target. If the boat occasionally steers off course, then you take action and correct it in order to head back towards your goal/target.

Caring for Your Health from One Doctor's Visit to the Next!

If you think that your health is solely the responsibility of your doctor, think again. It is estimated that an average visit with a doctor is no more than five minutes, and you may get to see your busy doctor once or twice per year. From visit to visit, things may go terribly wrong with your blood sugar, blood pressure, and your cholesterol. From visit to visit, your lifestyle habits may change, your weight may increase, your activity levels may drop, and you could have added, on a daily basis, several more hours of TV watching at the start of the "Game" season, accompanied by drinking enormous amounts of alcohol or soft drinks, munching on buttered popcorn, loads of chips and other salty snacks like pizza, hot dogs and the whole works. If you are a smoker you may have increased your smoking frequency at the start of the game season or due to stress. All of these actions will contribute to tipping your weight scale north, causing your blood sugar, blood pressure and cholesterol to go out of control and consequently raising your chances of major heart attacks or debilitating strokes all before your next doctor's visit.

Moreover, during that next visit, your doctor may, most likely, not be aware of all these changes; and if you don't provide him or her with your daily blood sugar and blood pressure results, he or she may inappropriately make an incorrect change to your treatment. Waiting for the next doctor's visit to find and correct a problem can be detrimental to your health, and it can mean the difference between life and death; this is, by far, an inaccurate and dangerous way to monitor your condition. Get ahead of the game, and prevent avoidable heart attacks or strokes or worse.

If you choose to remain in this situation, then this is no different than choosing, voluntarily, to be in that boat without navigation gear, embarking on a journey into oblivion.

Janet's Story Represents Millions of People with Diabetes: People Whose Condition Goes Unnoticed and Undiagnosed, and Who Quietly Suffer from Having Their Condition Slide Dangerously Out of Control

One day, during my pharmacy practice, one lady showed up to the pharmacy-counseling window, wanting to speak to the pharmacist. I went there and offered my assistance to Janet, as she introduced herself to me. Janet wanted some recommendations for leg pains she was having. She asked me, "Is Tylenol or Motrin better for leg pain?" However, before I was about to give a recommendation, I wanted to know more? Janet could not have been more than 55 years old, and she was overweight. So I probed further to understand the source of her leg pain. Janet replied that she had some numbness and tingling in her feet, and that she experienced pain after walking a short distance. She also complained of blurred vision. The symptoms Janet gave me were classic complications of uncontrolled diabetes, where the sugar had been high for quite some time, above the recommended levels of 110 mg/dl and had already started causing some damage to nerve endings and arteries, which were the reason for Janet's complaints.

Janet explained, further, that she was diagnosed with Type 2 Diabetes about three years prior, and she was under the impression that everything "was going okay" with her condition. Since I suspected that her blood sugar and various parameters were not under control, I went on to ask her about her sugar reading that morning; asking how frequently she monitored her sugar and what her last A1C level was. Of course, Janet replied, "I don't know what my last sugar reading was," let alone the A1C reading; she did not even know what A1C was, " The A1, what?" she replied. She was also clueless about her blood pressure and cholesterol readings.

However, she did tell me that the last time she was at the doctor's office, about 4 or 5 months prior, that the doctor had told her that everything was "OK." When I inquired about that "OK" reading, she said she forgot what it was, exactly, that he quoted her; but she did recall that her fasting sugar reading might have been about 140 or 150mg/dl. When I also inquired about her blood pressure, she likewise said that when she checked it last time at the pharmacy, "about a month ago," that it was "normal," about 140/90. She didn't remember the last cholesterol test she had taken, and she was not, then, taking any medications for cholesterol. She also revealed to me that she was on once-a-day Glyburide for blood sugar and a blood pressure pill.

When I inquired about the reason she did not monitor more frequently, she said, "My last monitor broke down about 6 months ago, and since my doctor always took my blood sugar reading at the clinic with every visit, about every 4 to 6 months then what do I need a monitor for." Janet's reality is a classic and sad story that keeps repeating itself, daily, with millions of people, just like Janet, who are headed down the path of real danger; this danger is churning inside them, all because: they are not monitoring properly, they are ignoring what the safe readings are, and they are making their health the responsibility of their doctor; most of all, they do not realize the real and immediate danger in which they have put themselves when their combined multiple risk factors spin out of control.

Janet and the millions like her are blindly navigating the journey of potentially dangerous enemies such as uncontrolled diabetes, high blood cholesterol, high blood pressure, and heart disease; Janet and these millions are ill-equipped, and their illness will compound several-fold, causing debilitating handicaps such as strokes, amputations and blindness, as well as other potentially fatal complications. Statistically speaking, it has been shown that about only 20-25% of diabetics monitor their sugar on a daily and consistent basis; due to this lack of monitoring, they become very likely candidates for suffering deadly complications that could simply have been averted. My pharmacist colleagues and I confirm this sad reality through our observations culled from our daily practice.

I realized, then, that I desperately needed to intervene and help Janet; surely, my advice did not consist of simply suggesting Tylenol or Advil for her leg pain. As I was speaking with Janet, my prescription load became backed up, and I had a couple of calls holding for me; however, in spite of all this, I managed to provide her with vital information about her condition in a brief manner. I asked her to come by the next day, when I had more pharmacy techs on the clock to help, freeing me up a bit so that I could spend more time with her.

In that brief moment, I explained to Janet that, since her sugar levels were out of whack, damage to her nervous system and blood vessels had started to occur, and "that" was the cause of her leg pain and blurred vision. I suggested to her to aim at a target of fasting-blood-sugar-level below 110 points, and a blood pressure target below 130/80, in order to stop further damage. I also advised Janet to contact her doctor immediately and have him reassess her diabetes and blood pressure medications, insisting that she have him perform a cholesterol check and put her on cholesterol medications ASAP and a baby Aspirin a day. I explained the importance of daily sugar monitoring and daily blood pressure monitoring. I told her that when she came by the next day, I would match her up with the proper blood sugar monitor, which would be the best investment she would ever make regarding her health.

In order to stabilize her blood sugar, I gave her brief tips (all the while, keeping her leg pain and limitation in mind) on how to increase her activity in several bouts of 5-10 minutes during each day, urged her to move away from being sedentary, as much as possible, and also gave her food tips to reduce her hunger and stabilize her blood sugar by raising her daily fiber intake; I told her to have, every day, 3 main meals with balanced portions and content, along with a couple of fruit snacks. I reminded her to make food selections that are lower in sugar and higher in fiber, such as: whole grain or rye breads, brown rice and pasta, beans, vegetables, salads. We also discussed, briefly, making balanced food choices as discussed in detail in Action Step 4 (Making Favorable Lifestyle Choices).

I saw the glare in Janet's eyes; she couldn't help but shake my hand as she thanked me for all the valuable information I gave her. She had told me that no one had ever taken the time to explain all of this to her. She promised to come back the next day so I could match her up with the right blood sugar monitor. Janet then took off, and I went back and tried to catch up with my pharmacy operation.

Matching Janet with a Blood Glucose Monitor

The next day, Janet showed up to the pharmacy and wanted me to match her with a good blood glucose monitor. I took into consideration her financial situation, keeping that in perspective, along with her manual and visual capacity to handle that matching monitor.

Janet told me that she did not want to mess with handling strips and also stated that she wanted a monitor with the least possible handling functions and to have the possibility of alternative site testing besides the fingers.

I advised her to get the "Accu-Check Compact" since the strips are in a drum, and when initially inserted into the machine, they get calibrated automatically with your intervention (One less step); Janet would not need to worry about calibrating the machine with each new batch of strips; and when ready to test blood, all she would have to do would be to push down a button to activate the machine; the machine automatically calibrates itself for the new strips, and also, the machine automatically draws out the strip and points the tip of the strip out in a ready position for the patient to drop the blood. The machine also has an extension for alternative blood drawing and requires a minute amount of blood to give an accurate reading.

As we started to talk about monitors, Janet confessed to me that the reason she did not want to mess with pricking her fingers is because she felt she was "clumsy," and every time she had to test her sugar, she would have to prick herself several times, waste lancets, and not get enough blood from her fingers, and then the strip would go bad before she would be able to draw enough blood from her fingers. "The whole thing would be a cumbersome and messy procedure, so I promised myself not to mess with testing my sugar anymore." Then it dawned on me, that I, as a professional, took these tasks for granted. I realized they might be more difficult and cumbersome for non-professionals, which could be a main barrier for people and make them not want to monitor. I told Janet that this machine would be a good match for her, since it's very efficient, it requires less maneuvering, requires very little blood, and the blood can be drawn from the less painful sites (such as the forearms and the hands, as well).

This section is for the curious only. If you have been drawing blood successfully from your fingers or other alternative sites, then you can skip this section.

Telling Janet about Proper Blood-Drawing Techniques and Instructions on How to Minimize Pain

I told Janet that I would tell her about the appropriate blood-drawing techniques so she could get enough blood, successfully, on the first attempt, and with much less pain! I suggested to Janet to follow the proper procedure for drawing blood from her finger:

The Finger-Pricking Technique:

1. Activate your machine and make sure the strip is out and ready to take up blood. This also applies to other people who have other machines; make sure the strip and machine are ready for the blood drop.

2. Draw more blood to the testing site by warming your hands with warm water, or by rubbing one hand with another for a few minutes, and by keeping them pointed downward. **Do not wipe fingers or alternative testing sites with alcohol** because as you prick your skin alcohol may be mixed with that drop of blood and may give a false reading.

3. Keep your hand down to your side, below your waistline for a few minutes.

4. Then hold the lancing device with one hand, while keeping your other hand below waistline; place the tip of the lancing device at the side of the tip of any finger, and not in the middle, because the center tip of the finger has more nerve endings and, consequently, will hurt more. When you have the lancing device on the side of the finger in the ready position, apply some pressure, and then release the lancer. Keep your hand down, and start performing milking-motion squeezes to your hand and to the finger that has been pricked. Stop the milking motion *up to the knuckle before last.*

5. Get the tip of the test strips (where the blood is uploaded) close to the blood drop that is coming out of your finger, and feed it to the strip, and keep it there until it takes enough blood.

6. The reading is displayed within a few seconds. Preferably write those readings down in a logbook, as a back up, in case the monitor's memory fails.

Alternative Pricking Sites:

- Likely alternative sites: the forearm, the upper arm, and both upper sides of the hands right above the palms, the thighs and calves. The skin in these areas is less sensitive than the fingers and, consequently, the procedure is less painful if you use these sites to prick.

- Rub the chosen site first, before pricking, for a couple of minutes in order to warm it up and get the blood running.

- Mount the forearm extension that comes with your meter of the lancing device; press it against your forearm skin or other chosen alternative site for a few seconds by applying pressure. This pressure that you apply on that site, before you release the lancing device, helps the blood to engorge, thus the blood will flow out more easily. Then press the lancing device release button. As the blood starts coming out, feed it to the strip as described above.

- Almost all lancing devices may have a pricking depth adjuster. If you have sensitive skin and don't do a lot of manual labor, then you might choose the least depth possible on that gauge. If, however, you have rough skin and you do a lot of labor with your hands and you have a lot of areas that are calloused, then you may need to adjust the device to a deeper pricking mode.

Important Lancing and Skin-Conditioning Tips:

- Practice proper techniques and you will be able to draw the desired amount of blood from the first attempt.
- Rotate the sites or the fingers being pricked to reduce skin irritation and to give enough time to that pricked site to heal.
- Most of the newer devices are designed to operate with small amounts of blood.
- Use daily moisturizing creams and Aloe Vera on the pricked sites to soothe and soften your skin. Also, drinking 6-8 glasses of water will help keep your skin soft.
- Use Hydrocortisone cream 3 times daily for a couple days, if the skin around the pricked sites becomes irritated or red.
- You may use some lancets more than once, but do not use them more than twice.
- Do not share used lancets with other people, and dispose of them properly in Sharps containers or tightly sealed used cans of juice or canned food receptacles.
- Find a monitor with which you are most comfortable. Refer to Table 2 on the next page for best picks.

Whichever monitor you decide to purchase, and whatever your financial status, **do invest in a monitor and do monitor your blood sugar daily. Buying a sugar monitor will be the best investment of your life.** Even if you have to borrow the money, you need to own a sugar monitor and monitor daily. Please also refer to the next upcoming section regarding the frequency of checking your blood sugar.

After we got the blood glucose monitoring issues out of the way, and Janet was content with the information she received, she went ahead and bought the machine, which I recommended, and she promised to start monitoring daily. But then other questions started popping up in her mind, and she started wondering about how she would make sense of all these sugar readings, and how relevant they were to her, and at what levels they should be at different times of day. She also asked me about A1C levels, blood pressure and cholesterol levels and proper monitoring frequency. She also inquired about check-ups for her feet, teeth and eyes. She wondered what check-ups are her responsibility and those that her doctor needed to suggest or monitor.

Table 2: Matching a Monitor with Your Specific Needs

Monitor Feature	Name	Quick Tips
For dexterity issues, no messing with strips and least maneuvering	• AccuCheck Compact • Ascensia Dex • Ascensia Breeze • Freestyle	• No calibration needed. • No adjusting of new strip batch number. • One-push button to activate system.
Hand tremors and vision problems	• AccuCheck Advantage • AccuCheck Comfort Curve	• Strips can be touched anywhere and still give an accurate reading. • Large screen display.
Vision problems	• AccuCheck Advantage • AccuCheck Comfort Curve • AccuCheck Voicemate	• Monitor can be activated by voice commands.
Alternative-site testing	• Freestyle • At Last • AccuCheck Ultra • AccuCheck Compact • Ultra Therasense • Most meters	• These monitors require the least amount of blood. • Most newer monitoring devices may have additional supplies for alternative-site testing.
Economical monitors	• Any retail chain store has its own cheaper brand. For instance, Wal-Mart's brand is called Ultima. • Accu-Check Active, • Prestige IQ	• The Ultima machine runs for about $15 or less. The cost of 50 strips is about $23; 100 strips $43-$44. • Strips for a house brand or a retail chain private label brand usually cost about 50% of the national leading brands, and they are all accurate. All monitors have equal accuracy. It is just the features that would match your special needs that differ.
Disposable monitors	• Sidekick	• This is a disposable blood sugar meter and strips, all in one unit. • The meter does not have to be coded. • Testing can be done on fingertips and forearms. • Requires a tiny amount of blood. • Once all 50 strips are used up, the whole system needs to be thrown away. • Does not have memory. • It cost about $35 for every 50 tests.

Janet brought up very interesting and crucial points. I was delighted with her level of interest and all the inquiries she had and voiced; this shows that she is becoming an active participant in her health and well being.

I told Janet that her health was solely her responsibility and no one else's. I also said that our health is the most important gift that God has given us, and that we have the ultimate responsibility of protecting it. If her health is not good, then nothing else matters and she will not be able to enjoy life, no matter how much money she has and no matter how many castles she owns.

As a start, I pointed Janet to the table below which reveals all the crucial parameters listed conveniently in one section, which she would need to keep up with and act upon. Her and ALL other diabetics need to get familiar with the lifesaving information included in the following table.

The information listed in Table 3 on the next page is based on recommendations from the American Diabetes Association, World Health Organization, and other reliable and reputable health organizations.

Janet's Inquiries

"How High or Low Should My Sugar Level Be, and Why Is It So Important to Keep It There?"

QUESTION: Janet wondered why it was so important to keep her fasting-morning-sugar below 110, and the evening sugar reading, which is about 2 hours after lunch and before dinner or any snack, should be below 145.

ANSWER: **First off, Janet, did you notice that in each of the categories in the far right boxes in the table above, entitled, "What Should I Do?" how it constantly repeats, "Keep your sugar under control"? That very necessary step is listed in each of those far right-hand boxes. No, this not a typographical error either. *The truth is that "keeping your sugar under control" is at the heart of keeping your diabetes under control.* Now, you know what "under control" means; just look at the table above. If you bring your sugar down to these levels that I listed in the table, then this may help to a great extent all your other levels to come down, including your triglyceride and blood pressure**

Table 3: The Compass Table of the Various Crucial Parameters That Every Diabetic Must Know and Monitor in Order to Navigate to Safety*

What to monitor?	Whose responsibility?	How often?	What it should be?	What should I do?
Your Eyes	Make the appointment with your eye doctor	Eye exam at the doctor's office every 6-12 months	20/20	Keep sugar under control
Blood Sugar	• Totally yours.	If using oral medication: • At least once in the AM while fasting, preferably another one 2 hours after lunch. If using insulin: • Before each injection and each morning before eating and at bedtime.	"Under Control" is: • **Morning before eating: below 110 and above 70 mg/dl.** • **Mid afternoon: 2 hours after lunch and before a snack: below 145.**	**Keep your sugar "under control":** • Own a sugar monitor; monitor your sugar, record your reading, compare to "Under control" levels and show your doctor. • Take medications as prescribed. • Start PRACTICING to make favorable lifestyle choices. (See Action Step 4 for details).
HbA1C or A1C	• The doctor's & yours. • You can now buy A1C monitor OTC. It is called "A1C Now" (and is inexpensive).	• Once every 3 months.	**Between 6 to below 7%.**	• Keep your sugar "under control." • Request the doctor to take it every 3 months. • Remember every 1% drop of A1C will reduce your chance of blindness and nerve damage by 35%.
Feet	• Yours. If you have a spouse or family member have them help you if you have physical limitations.	• Once every night. • Go through every inch of your feet and toes with the help of a mirror if by yourself.	• Skin should be clear with no scratches, blisters, rashes or any injuries. • You should have full sensation in your feet and legs. If your sugar is "under control" you will not have numbness, tingling or pain in your feet due to nerve damage. If you already have numbness and pain, then bringing your sugar "under control" will prevent further damage.	**Keep your sugar "under control":** • Maintain proper foot hygiene. • If there is any small cut, blister or damage to skin, or any numbness or tingling, contact your doctor right away; do not wait! • Apply moisturizing creams DAILY. Check the Diabetes section at your local pharmacy for various brands of aggressive foot creams. • Break in new shoes gradually over 3 weeks (2 hours a day & wear other broken-in shoes to work.

*NOTE: Details about each of these parameters are discussed beginning on page 60.

The Vital Importance of Monitoring...Treatment...Prevention

Table 3: *Cont.*

What to monitor?	Whose responsibility?	How often?	What should it be?	What should I do?
Cholesterol Total cholesterol LDL (Bad) HDL (Good) Triglyceride	• Your responsibility to remind your doctor to take it.	• If taking cholesterol medication, your doctor should request a blood test every 3 months for the first year, then every 6 months, thereafter. • If not taking medications for cholesterol then you should in order to keep your levels aggressively low as indicated in the next column.	"Under Control" is Total Cholesterol: • Below 135. LDL: • Below 100. HDL: • Over 40 (men). • Over 50 (women). Triglyceride: • Below 150.	Keep your sugar "under control." • Aim at keeping cholesterol within these limits and you will be safe. • Take medications daily as prescribed. • Keep a copy of cholesterol test issued by doctor, and compare levels listed there to previous readings. • If not taking medications, and your readings are above these levels, then call your doctor **NOW** and get on medications!
Blood Pressure	• Yours and your doctor's.	• Every morning or at least 4–5 times a week (see below for proper measurement technique).	"Under Control" is: • Below 130/80.	Keep your sugar "under control." • Monitor & record dates & show doctor your recorded numbers in your journal. • If consistently above 130/80, let doctor know immediately and don't wait to the next appointment or you may be in danger.
Dental Check-up	• Yours to make it to your dentist appointment.	• Twice a year.	• Your teeth and gums should be clear of any disease, infections or bleeding.	Keep your sugar "under control." • Keep good oral hygiene. • Floss after meals and at night. Brush every morning and after flossing, at night.

levels. All else becomes okay, and you move away from danger, and your risk of infections is reduced; also greatly reduced are the chances of damage to your nervous system, need for amputations, blindness, kidney damage, heart attacks and strokes. So that's why "Keep your sugar under control" is there so often!

Secondly, Janet, the American Diabetes Association, as a result of several landmark trials such as the "UKPDS" and "DCCT," recommends that keeping tight sugar control at the levels mentioned in the table above can drastically reduce these complications. All it simply takes to spare your organs and your limbs from destruction is a blood sugar monitor that tells you what your daily sugar levels are, just like the navigation system on that boat, you need this navigation system to guide you out of an impending wreck.

Finally, Janet, your compass to safety includes: monitoring your sugar with the sugar monitor machine; taking your medications on a regular basis as prescribed; developing the habits of making favorable lifestyle choices; and if you notice any increase in these levels, let your doctor know immediately, so he or she can intervene appropriately and in a timely fashion. That's all. Remember, as your sugar levels rise and remain above these recommended levels, it is slowly but surely creating irreversible damage to your internal organs. Precious years can unduly be slashed from your lifespan. However, if you take these very simple actions, as discussed in this paragraph, and if you aim at keeping your sugar levels in check as in that table, then you can reap the priceless rewards of averting complications, achieving a natural lifespan and enjoying the ultimate quality of life.

Janet exclaimed, "I didn't realize it was that simple! I was told that I was okay as long as my sugar level was below 150 or 160 and my blood pressure at 150/90, but I guess your information is more up-to-date. I will definitely stick with what you are telling me."

"What Is 'A1C' and How Relevant Is It to My Diabetes Control?" Janet Asks

"You told me my A1C should be between 6 or 7%. Why is that reading so important? And how should I monitor it, and how frequent should that reading be taken"? Janet asked.

"Janet, A1C, or what used to be referred to as HbA1C, is a measurement of the average glucose amount in your red blood cells over the last 3 months; it's a very considerable measurement. Your doctor should do this reading every 3 months. The desired level of the A1C should be below 7% and ideally closer to 6%. However, there is now an A1C test available over-the-counter that you can purchase from any retail chain. It's called "A1C Now" and allows you to take that reading at home very inexpensively at a cost of about $10-$15 per test every 3 months."

"Also, Janet, studies have revealed that the A1C parameter is a very powerful indicator of how well your diabetes is doing. Every 1% rise of your A1C over 7% will raise your chances of having all kinds of complications such as blindness, amputations, neuropathy (the tingling feeling, nerve ending damage and pain and loss of sensation in your feet and hands), by a whopping 35%. Also tight sugar control decreases drastically the incidence of kidney damage. You realize now that the tingling you have been experiencing in your feet is because you have suffered some nerve damage, neuropathy. This occurred due to your consistently elevated blood sugar level. On the other hand, as your blood sugar starts dropping to below 110 in a fasting state, then further nerve damage can and will stop and even your current leg pain may improve.

"So Janet, this is one additional reason why you should become involved in your health and get your diabetes under control."

"Why Is It So Important for Me to Check My Feet DAILY?"

I had asked Janet whether she had been checking her feet daily for any cuts or blisters. She replied, "No, why would I?" I told Janet that since she had diabetes, she would have a hard time fighting off infections, and that cuts, blisters, or burns to her skin, especially in her feet, would also pose problems; besides which, since she had diabetes, she would have a tendency to have dry skin due to poor circulation. The dryness could then cause cracks in her feet, and ulcers could potentially form; and since she mentioned she had been experiencing tingling and numbness in her feet, consequently, this means it is possible she could have lost some sensory perception there and may not know or feel that she had any cuts or blisters in the foot area unless she visually inspected her feet on a daily basis. I also told Janet, that in the United States alone, up to 60% or more of all leg and partial limb amputations, yearly, are due to diabetes.

By far, these leg amputations can be prevented if diabetics keep their sugar under control. "By God, Janet, can you imagine not being able to walk or get around to do your daily chores at your young age?" **Everyone with diabetes has the power to change his or**

her lives for the better. It is truly easy. Anybody can keep his or her diabetic condition under control. I reminded Janet that any time she discovered any blister or cut in her feet, to let her doctor know immediately. She should not wait. During my practice, I have counseled people who had cuts and blisters on their feet for several weeks and who did not seek medical treatment for them. These are the very same seeds, which begin the trauma that later fully develops into leg, toe and limb amputations. **At the first sign of cuts or blisters to the feet, DO NOT SELF TREAT IT but seek immediate medical treatment.**

The Story of a Diabetic Employee Who Comes Limping From a Foot Ulcer to the Pharmacy

I have come across several situations where I have counseled people who had diabetes and people who had foot ulcers and cuts for quite sometime, and them not having sought immediate medical attention. In one instance, I was working at a retail pharmacy, and one of the employees came limping to the pharmacy-counseling window. He asked me for my advice about a topical cream that he could apply on a foot wound. After inquiring further, I learned that he had diabetes and that he had been trying to break into his new shoes (which was the cause for the blisters on his feet). When I inquired about how long that ulcer had been there, he told me it had been there for about three weeks; he also mentioned that he'd tried to self-treat it, but he noticed it getting worse. Despite this fact, he did not yet "see a need" to contact his doctor. My advice to him, at that time, was to go directly to the emergency room or to his doctor and receive immediate medical attention.

He didn't seem to be in a hurry or realize the predicament in which he'd placed himself. He mentioned to me that he could not take off work unless he had a "true medical emergency." I replied to him, "This is a real medical emergency, and unless you seek treatment right away, you could very well be facing the grave danger of losing your leg!" I learned that the next day, he went on to have his foot diagnosed and was immediately put on aggressive antibiotic treatment. I had seen this man regularly for several months since then, and the ulcer to his foot had not yet healed; actually, it had taken a turn for the worse, even though he had been on continuous use of antibiotics. What compounded the problem was that his blood sugar was not under control. I am not sure of the outcome to his leg since I relocated to another store. I fear he might have eventually ended up with an amputation.

I pointed out to Janet that it was very important for her to check her feet daily, in order to avoid ending up like that employee. I instructed her, that if she had no one available to help her check her foot area, that she could then use a mirror with an extended arm to check every inch of her feet on a daily basis. I also added that, right after she checks her feet is the best time to apply an aggressive moisturizer to both her feet and hands on a daily basis; this keeps the skin well-conditioned, thus reducing incidents and complications. I also suggested she puts some foot powder before she wore her shoes to keep her feet dry; this prevents fungal infections. The feet contain the highest number of sweat glands, and moisture is the breeding ground for fungus, which can highly complicate matters for a diabetic, and cause skin and toe nail fungal which could be challenging to treat.

I also suggested to her that she break in new shoes "gradually." The way to do so is by wearing the new shoe a couple of hours each day, then switch to the comfortable shoes. I told her that every few days, she could increase the amount of time she wore that new shoe by an hour or two; in about three weeks the skin on her feet may be able to handle that new pair all day long, without any problems.

"How Frequently Should I Have My Eyes And Teeth Checked?" Asked Janet

Let's Start with Eye Care Tips

It is recommended by the American Diabetes Association that diabetics have at least one eye examination per year (if the diabetes is under control); if not, then once every 6 months. **If you are experiencing blurred vision, chances are that your sugar is out of control, thus starting to destroy the small blood vessels in your eyes and affecting your vision.** If this problem is not addressed soon, then you can go blind. I reminded Janet that diabetes is the leading cause of blindness among adults. It does not have to be that way! Blindness can be prevented! Imagine spending the rest of your life in darkness, not being able to see your grandchildren or other loved ones, not being able to see and make your way around, not being able to drive or witness the beauty of this world. Everybody who has diabetes has all the power to change the course of their future and age gracefully, instead of tragically, by keeping their diabetes under control.

Next, Let's Talk about Tooth Care

As I mentioned earlier to Janet, high blood sugar levels damage blood vessels and nerve cells; high blood sugar levels also weaken your immunity and reduce the capacity of your white blood cells and other immune cells to capture and destroy invading bacteria/organisms. Consequently, you will have a much higher chance of having infections in your gums and teeth, leading to periodontal disease. As a consequence of these infections, tooth loss may occur at a much higher rate for those whose blood sugar levels are out of control, as opposed to those who keep their sugar under control. Also, painful chewing may result from these infections, leading you to select foods that are not ideal for your diabetic condition.

After making the above comments to Janet, she asked, "So, am I doomed?"

"Not at all," I replied. You can be in full control, provided that you:

1. Get your sugar levels "under control" and by informing your diabetes doctor of high sugar levels immediately.

2. Get in touch with your dentist as soon as you experience one or more of the following situations:

    - Bleeding gums
    - Toothache
    - Mouth sores
    - Loose teeth
    - Poorly fitted dentures

And don't forget to inform your dentist that you have diabetes.

3. Perform these routine actions:

    a. Schedule a dental cleaning and checkup twice a year.

    b. Be diligent about dental hygiene:

    - Brush gently, all sides of your teeth, in the morning and before bedtime (after flossing). Flossing helps remove food lodged between your teeth which otherwise can create infectious bacteria that infects your teeth and gums.

    - Brush your tongue to remove infection-causing bacteria.

    - Limit the consumption of simple sugars, such as candy and sweetened chocolate, as they can turn within a short period of time to an acid that can cause tooth decay, let alone shoot up your blood sugar and cause you to be hungry in about 30 minutes. In the event that you consume a small portion of candy, chew a sugar free gum immediately afterwards to draw saliva to your mouth; this can neutralize the effects of that acid. or swish with drinking water, then spit or swallow it. You can also swish with any over-the-counter mouthwashes.

By taking these precautionary measures, you can ensure having healthy teeth, gums, and a beautiful smile.

CHOLESTEROL

How Important is Cholesterol Control, What Are the New Recommended Cholesterol Levels, and What Medications Are Available to Treat High Cholesterol?

I proceeded to ask Janet about her cholesterol and wondered when the last time was that her doctor requested a cholesterol test for her. She told me that her cholesterol level was borderline, and reiterated that her doctor did not seem to be worried. "It is funny you asked," Janet replied, "being that I brought a copy of my cholesterol test with me." I immediately congratulated her for keeping a copy of her cholesterol results (and everyone should, because you're paying for it; and you get to compare progress of your cholesterol results from one test to the next). **The overwhelming majority of people ignore their current cholesterol levels and where they should be.**

For a diabetic, THE THREE MOST CRUCIAL PARAMETERS to keep "under control" are:

1. Blood sugar
2. Cholesterol
3. Blood pressure

Keep them at bay, as recommended in the above table, and be safe.

I began to look at the test results that Janet had brought me; her cholesterol profile had a total cholesterol level of 211 mg/dl: her LDL (bad cholesterol) was at 142; her HDL (good cholesterol) was at 36; and her triglycerides were at 228. Now let's compare these readings with the recommended levels in the table above or the recommendations of the American Diabetes Association.

It is recommended that your total cholesterol should be below 135; your bad cholesterol, (LDL) below 100; the good cholesterol (HDL) above 50; and the triglycerides to be below 150, in order to avoid heart and artery disease and all other diabetes complications, which, you should by now know by heart.

"So if you compare your reading to what is recommended, Janet, you are way off on all of these parameters," I remarked. "Since, initially, you told me that you have a family history of cholesterol problems on both your paternal and maternal side, and since you told me that your dad suffered a heart attack a few years back, I must tell you that if you don't get on medications immediately to lower your cholesterol levels, you can be at a much-increased risk for a heart attack or stroke!"

Nowadays, more recent studies have surfaced and have shown the drastic benefits to diabetics in preventing imminent heart attacks when their cholesterol readings are kept significantly low.

It is recommended that all people who have diabetes be on cholesterol medication, preferably the "Statins" (which will be discussed later in this section), to aggressively bring to recommended levels, as in the table above, all the cholesterol parameters in order to avoid danger. The landmark studies named "UKPDS" and "DCCT" have shown that the risk of developing heart attacks and strokes drop considerably if cholesterol and blood pressure levels drop to recommended levels. This is achieved by both taking medications and making favorable lifestyle choices.

"What I suggest to you, Janet is to contact your doctor and ask him/her to get you started on a "Statin" cholesterol medication now. Once your cholesterol is brought down to the recommended levels, you will have a new lease on life."

Janet replied inquisitively and with a sigh, "More medications? There must be something terribly wrong with me. How long will I have to take these cholesterol pills?"

I urged Janet not to be stigmatized by the fact that she would be taking more medications; I told her that her only worry should be to make sure that her cholesterol levels do not remain out of balance, which drastically increases her risk of heart attacks or strokes. Taking medications to keep life threatening conditions under control will be a lifesaver! **Medications, when needed, should be construed as a good and positive thing.** "Only by lowering your cholesterol aggressively, can you have a new lease on life; the statistics don't lie," I told her. "**Just think of it as an additional vitamin pill that will**

literally save your life!" I also urged Janet to contact her doctor ASAP, so she could get started on cholesterol medication.

MUST READ: I urge Janet and everyone else who suffers from chronic conditions: Think of medications as lifesavers, not as detriments. The benefits of medications to treat chronic conditions such as diabetes, cholesterol, heart disease and blood pressure, far outweigh any short-lived side effects. If you have any concerns about side effects or drug interactions, then speak with your pharmacist or doctor before making any decisions about stopping your treatment or changing your dosage amount or dosage times. (Have I stressed this point enough already? I will mention it more, throughout, because during my practice I saw and continue to see this problem happening frequently: people making personal decisions to stop their medications or take them differently than prescribed, which causes conditions to worsen leading to unnecessary life-threatening complications). The most important factor here should be to keep your condition under control by taking medications as prescribed, by making favorable lifestyle choices, and by not having a stigma about taking medications.

Cholesterol Medications

NOTE: This section is for the curious only. You may read about the drugs you are currently taking. If you wish to skip, you can go to the next section and learn about blood pressure.

WHICH CHOLESTEROL MEDICATIONS ARE AVAILABLE AND WHAT YOU SHOULD KNOW ABOUT THEM

WARNING: As a general rule, when taking any medications and if you are allergic to its content and start experiencing very rare but serious reactions such as difficulty swallowing, difficulty breathing, and/or swelling of the tongue, throat or lips then stop that medication and immediately call emergency services. You could also have someone take you to the emergency room of the closest hospital immediately, and get medical treatment. These are rare allergic reactions, but they can be life-threatening if not immediately treated.

THE FIRST GROUP OF CHOLESTEROL-LOWERING DRUGS

This line of cholesterol-lowering medication, which would be ideal for Janet and other diabetics, is referred to as "the Statins." This group of medication is very aggressive in lowering bad cholesterol (LDL) by up to 60% or more, and triglycerides by up to 40% or more, and by raising heart-protective good cholesterol (HDL) by up to 40% or more. Some of the medications available in this group are:

Statins:

- Altoprev
- Crestor
- Lipitor
- Lescol
- Mevacor (cheaper and equally effective generic is available)
- Pravachol (cheaper and equally effective generic is available)
- Zocor (cheaper and equally effective generic is available)

How Do They Work?

In general, these medications are most effective in the evening, since they target the liver's capacity to produce cholesterol, which happens at night. However, Pravacol, Crestor, and Lipitor can be taken at any time during the day. Your doctor will select the appropriate medication and dose that is best suited for you.

Possible Side Effects

Some mild and short-lived side effects such as:

- Nausea
- Stomach upset
- Dry mouth
- Momentary sleep disturbances
- And liver function may be affected

Most importantly, **a rare but serious side effect can occur at any time while on these medications, requiring your attention and immediate action.** While on these Statins, if at any time during the course of your treatment, you develop:

- General muscle or bone pain and/or weakness or tenderness to any muscles in your body, (as a whole or in part) to any muscle groups, such as your leg or back or any other parts of your body, then stop taking the medication and contact your doctor as soon as possible and let him or her know.

All your doctor has to do is change your medication, and this condition called "Rhabdomyolysis," which means the breakdown of your body muscles, is reversible. If this condition develops and you keep taking this medication, then general muscle breakdown is expedited and total kidney failure and other complications may ensue. Your doctor may require a blood test from you to confirm this finding with a parameter named "CPK." The normal blood level of this parameter should be approximately 170 mg/dl. You need not panic about this medicine, because Rhabdomyolysis is a rare occurrence.

Just watch for the signs just mentioned and remembers that the benefits of these medications far outweigh the consequences, and I confirm to you that these medications are LIFESAVERS. Virtually every diabetic can benefit from the "Statins" or other cholesterol-lowering medications; and remember that by aggressively lowering your total cholesterol to below 135 mg/dl, you will be in a much safer place.

Monitoring Required from Your Doctor while on These Medications

For the first year that you are on these medications, your doctor should require a blood test from you every 3 months to check out your liver function and to monitor how well the medication is lowering your cholesterol. After 1 year, then once every 6 months is appropriate to check your blood work. Why have a blood test:

1. To monitor the effect of the medication on your cholesterol and keep track of your cholesterol readings.
2. To monitor your liver function.
3. To monitor for "CPK" (a reading which may show the signs of that rare but potential side effect that affects your muscles while on the "Statins").

What Foods to Avoid while on These Medications

Do not combine grapefruit juices or the fruit itself with the "Statin" family because it may raise the level of such medications in your blood and by doing so it increases the occurrence chances of that rare muscle problem.

Medications NOT to Combine with the "Statins"

Antibiotics such as:

- Erythromycin
- Levaquin
- Cipro
- Nizoral
- Sporanox
- Ketek
- Zpack
- Biaxin

Or:

- Over-the-counter Tagamet (for stomach acid)
- Allopurinol
- Valproic Acid

These should not be combined with Statins, as they may raise the chances of that rare muscle problem. While on these Antibiotics, you need to stop the Statins and resume them only after the antibiotic treatment is over. Instead of Tagamet, choose Pepcid or Zantac. About the other drugs, your doctor will make the decision about changing either treatments or doses.

On the other hand, if you are on drugs such as:

- Dilantin
- Tegretol
- Phenobarbital
- Rifampin

Then the effect of the Statins may be lowered, and your doctor should regulate the dosages of each of these medications.

Also, do not combine these or any others drugs within 2 hours of over-the-counter stomach acid reducers known as antacids. These include:

- Maalox
- Mylanta
- Peptobismol
- Tums
- Other similar products in this category

These antacids may lower the absorption of other drugs, making them less effective.

Who Should NOT Take the Statin Medications?

- Women who are pregnant, nursing or planning to become pregnant.
- People who have any type of muscle degeneration/disease.

- People who have inadequate kidney and/or liver function or who have kidney and/or liver failure.

THE SECOND GROUP OF CHOLESTEROL-LOWERING DRUGS

Niacin (Vitamin B3): A medication which lowers total cholesterol, bad cholesterol and is aggressive in increasing the good cholesterol.

Janet, if your good cholesterol is below 40, and if for some reason you cannot take any of the "Statins" or cannot afford them, then Niaspan (prescription drug), or Niacin or Slo-Niacin (both over-the-counter), all have the same active ingredient (Niacin or Vitamin B3), are good alternatives. This medication will increase your good cholesterol (HDL) and will also lower your bad cholesterol (LDL), as well as lower your triglycerides, but not to the extent of the Statins. Niacin works by reducing your body's capacity to produce cholesterol, but in a different way than the Statins.

<u>**Possible Side Effects**</u>:
- Facial flushing
- Dizziness
- Muscle pain
- Palpitations
- Increase in blood sugar

Therefore, monitoring your blood sugar daily, as mentioned before, will help you detect any fluctuation in your blood sugar when you start this medication. **Flushing** may be remedied by taking about 81 to 160 milligrams of aspirin about 30 minutes before taking this medication. Since you should be taking aspirin anyway, and if you are taking this medication to lower cholesterol, the best time to take your aspirin would be right before taking this medication.

What Your Doctor Should Monitor

Your doctor should require a blood test performed every 3 months, just like he requires for the Statins; this blood test's purpose is to look for how well it's working on your cholesterol, as well as to monitor your liver function. If Niacin is combined with a Statin drug for a further cholesterol lowering effect, then chances are higher for that rare but potential problem of muscle aches and pain. Then again, let your doctor know of any such occurrences.

The Third Group of Cholesterol-Lowering Drugs

Fibrates: An aggressive group of medications that treat high triglycerides.

Now, Janet, if you have high triglyceride levels above 150 mg/dl, then I will mention again that first, it is vital that your sugar be dropped to recommended levels, and then your triglyceride level may drop lower as well.

To drop your triglycerides further, there is a group of medications named "Fibrates" which aggressively lower your triglyceride level. Namely, there is Lopid (available in generic form, Gemfibrozil), and also Tricor and other Fibrates, now available on the market.

Fibrates work by ridding your body of substances that cause the formation of triglycerides and by reducing their production. Fibrates also lower your total bad cholesterol (LDL) and raise your good cholesterol (HDL). Fibrates can be administered along with the Statins to aggressively lower your triglycerides and cholesterol even further.

Possible Side Effects

Some mild and transient side effects can occur such as:
- Stomach disturbances
- Indigestion
- Nausea
- Flatulence
- Dizziness
- Slight weight gain
- Muscle aches
- Dizziness
- Sleep disturbances
- A mild rash

When used with Statins, Lopid (Gemfibrozil) increases the chance of that rare side effect which the "Statins" can cause to your muscles; but the newer Fibrates, such as Tricor, have much less potential of causing that problem.

What Your Doctor Should Monitor for

Your doctor needs to request a blood work-up from you every 3 months for the first year while you are on this medication; and he/she needs to order liver function tests and total cholesterol tests in order to monitor for liver function and for how well this drug is working on your cholesterol and triglycerides.

Who Should NOT Take this Medication?

People who have kidney, liver and gallbladder diseases should NOT take these medications.

The Fourth Group of Cholesterol-Lowering Drugs

Two potential cholesterol-lowering medications named Zetia and Vytorin have been added lately to the arsenal of life-saving medications to reduce cholesterol.

Zetia: How Does It Work?

Zetia is the first to a new class of cholesterol-lowering medications. Zetia, alone, modestly reduces your total cholesterol by about 13% and your bad cholesterol (LDL) by 20%, also reducing your triglyceride by 8%. Zetia will raise your good cholesterol (HDL) by no more than 3 or 4%. Zetia works by preventing the absorption of cholesterol from your small intestines, consequently reducing how much cholesterol reaches your blood and your liver.

What Are Possible Side Effects?

Zetia is generally well-tolerated. Some people may experience, momentarily, some:

- Abdominal discomfort
- Diarrhea
- Fatigue
- Mild muscle aches

If you are sensitive to this medication, the first sign would be rash, and you must stop taking the medication.

Zetia is generally combined with other medications in the Statins family. The cholesterol-lowering effects of such a combination more than doubles. Since the combination of Zetia and a "Statin" is so powerful, one company put out both of them in one drug, Vytorin.

Vytorin: How Does It Work?

Vytorin is a powerful combination of Zetia and Zocor in one pill. This is a great benefit, in terms of combining two classes of cholesterol-lowering drugs in one pill, and it is also convenient.

The cholesterol lowering effect more than doubles when two products that works in different ways to reduce cholesterol (such as Zetia and Zocor) are combined. Zetia prevents cholesterol absorption from food, and Zocor prevents your liver from producing cholesterol. The combined benefit of Vytorin is a whopping reduction of up to 42% in total cholesterol, 60% reduction of bad cholesterol (LDL), and 32% reduction in triglycerides, as well as an 8% elevation in good cholesterol (HDL).

What You Should Know about Vytorin

- Your doctor will decide what medications to put you on and at what dose.
- Take Vytorin in the evening or at bedtime, because it has a member of the "Statin" that is most effective at night.
- Take on a regular basis every evening, and do not change the dosage or frequency of how you take it without consulting your doctor.
- Your doctor will have to require a blood test every 3 months for the first year. For more details on this issue review the "Statins" and " Zetia."

Omacor: How Does It Work?

Omacor is one of the most recent medications on the market for treating high triglycerides. This drug is ideal for people who have triglycerides above 500 mg/dl, such as those with uncontrolled diabetes, who for some reason cannot tolerate other medications or who have experienced poor results with other medications that were unsuccessful in reducing their triglyceride levels. Omacor is the only FDA approved drug that contains fish oil, and is available by prescription only.

Other conditions, such as thyroid disorders, may raise triglycerides. Other drugs such as the blood pressure medications, Beta Blockers, water pills such as Hydrochlorothiazide and estrogen pills may all raise triglyceride levels.

Possible Side Effects

Fish oils may have side effects such as:
- Burping
- Flu-like effects
- Upset stomach
- Rash
- Change in taste

If somebody is taking blood thinning medication such as:

- Coumadin
- Plavix
- Aspirin
- Or any others

They need to monitor their blood flow periodically, because Omacor can cause further thinning of the blood. Omacor should be stopped after 2-3 months if it cannot produce the desired results. The dose of Omacor is 4 capsules of 1 gram each to be taken as a single dose or twice a day with meals.

COMBINATION DRUGS TO LOWER CHOLESTEROL

Finally, a cholesterol combination drug that combines Niacin and a Statin drug called Mevacor are now available in a one-pill form called Advicor. It combines two powerful cholesterol- lowering drugs that work in different manners in aggressively reducing cholesterol, all with the convenience of taking only one pill at night.

Caduet is another combination of a "Statin" drug named Lipitor and a blood pressure medication called Norvasc. This is a clever combination to combine a blood pressure-lowering medication along with a blood cholesterol-lowering medication all in the convenience of taking one pill a day that lowers both.

It is imperative to mention again that all cholesterol medications are always prescribed to lower cholesterol (and they work best when you make favorable lifestyle choices and building habits of making balanced food choices and raising the level of activity daily). If you are a smoker, it is needless to say that you need to quit smoking as soon as possible, because smoking is a main contributor to heart disease along with a long list of other deadly ailments; it is the number one killer in the United States and causes your cholesterol parameters to go out of whack. So taking medications on a regular basis, making favorable lifestyle choices, stopping tobacco dependence, and reducing your stress levels are your only ticket to averting major health catastrophes and having peace of mind and experiencing the best quality of life.

Blood Pressure

How Can Blood Pressure Be Controlled in Someone Who Has Diabetes? And What Is the Ideal Blood Pressure Reading?

This is the third and one of the most important factors to keep under control. We had mentioned first, that in order for somebody who has diabetes to have a life free of complications and have a natural lifespan, he or she must keep three things "under control." The first and second is to keep sugar and cholesterol "under control," as we have already discussed. Thirdly, you must **keep your blood pressure "under control," making sure it is below 130/80; thus avoiding heart attacks and strokes that could shatter your life.**

Janet asked me, "Why is it so important to keep my blood pressure under control? I was under the impression that a blood pressure reading of 140 to 150 over 90 or 95 is OK. Is that true?"

I told Janet that having **uncontrolled cholesterol and blood pressure levels raise her chances 4-fold of having heart disease, heart attacks, and disease of the arteries (Atherosclerosis). Blood pressure affects up to a staggering 73% of people with diabetes; also, up to a whopping 75% of diabetic complications are caused by high blood pressure. In fact, studies have shown that more than half the people diagnosed with diabetes have had Atherosclerosis for years or decades prior to their diagnosis of it. By the way, smoking is a major cause of this disease as well. Unfortunately, the disease of the arteries is responsible for claiming the lives of more than 65% of all people who have diabetes. This is very disturbing and alarming, especially that the major threats of high blood pressure and cholesterol are controllable and can be avoided and even may be reversed in some cases.**

I responded to Janet's question, "First of all, your blood pressure, which is currently about 145 over 90 or 95 is elevated, according to today's standards. It is recommended by the American Diabetes Association, that in order to avert major heart attacks and strokes, people with diabetes should keep their blood pressure below 130/80. The medications your doctor wisely prescribed for your blood pressure is called Lisinopril/ HCTZ 20/12.5 mg, belongs to a class of blood pressure medications called ACE Inhibitors, which have been shown to not only be very effective in reducing your blood pressure but also to protect your heart and kidneys from further complications. Also combined to that medication is a water pill which is also an effective way to treat your blood pressure and which we will discuss later in this section.

The ACE Inhibitors' class of blood pressure-lowering medication, along with the other groups of drugs such as the ARB drugs, the water pills and Beta Blockers, which we will discuss in a more detailed fashion a little later on in this section, are truly lifesaving. Yes, you may have to take these blood pressure medications permanently, but you must think of it as the best thing that ever happened to you, since all of these medications do not have any irreversible long-term side effects and will help you lower your blood pressure to a safe zone and avert debilitating, if not fatal, heart attacks and strokes. As I've suggested before, just think of this as a multivitamin that you are taking on a daily basis, and look for the additional details on the medicine/s later on in this section.

Janet, your responsibility is to help your doctor lower your blood pressure. How? By YOU MAKING THE DECISION to begin adopting favorable lifestyle choices as of TODAY increase your activity while waiting for your prescription that we are filling. Instead of sitting down, you should walk around the store until we finish filling your prescriptions. Every minute of activity helps. Get your blood moving and burn more energy as you move. Also, you need to make favorable food choices and follow the recommendations about lifestyle changes that are discussed in detail in Action Step 4. **Remember this magic number, Janet: 130/80 or below should be your ideal blood pressure as recommended by the American Diabetes Association and the American Heart Association.**

The only way you can know that your blood pressure is down is by monitoring your blood pressure on a daily basis or at least 4-5 times a week. Record these readings along with the date you took them, and keep track of them this way, in a log or journal. Then, inform your doctor if your blood pressure remains consistently above 130/80. Also, you need to realize that as you are starting a new blood pressure medication, it might take a week or two before you can see the maximum benefit being achieved. **However, if you, at any time, have an alarming high blood pressure rate, one that climbs above 170 or 180 over 110, do not wait 2 or 3 weeks before you notify your doctor. Call him and let him know right away, or call emergency assistance right away and get your blood pressure as close as possible to this magic number, 130/80.** Otherwise, you might be at risk of having a stroke or a heart attack.

Several landmark studies, such as the "UKPDS," shows that with every 10 point drop in your blood pressure:

- Your chances of having any diabetic complications drops by 12%.
- Your chances of having a heart attack drops by 11%.
- Your chances of going blind or having any kidney problems drops by 13%.
- This blood pressure reduction also reduces your mortality rate by 15%.

These amazing crystal-clear facts show that, just by reducing your blood pressure by a mere 10 points, you reap all these amazing benefits; and the closer you bring your blood pressure to below 130/80, you are reducing your chances of deadly complications, so much so, that they become comparable to someone who does not have diabetes or any chronic conditions. This is doable, Janet. It can be achieved. There is an arsenal of medications and endless categories of blood pressure lowering medications out there, which can help you, succeed in keeping your diabetes at bay. Taking the appropriate blood pressure medications and doses EVERY DAY, as prescribed by your doctor, along with lifestyle changes is your magic formula to safety and peace of mind.

If you have chronic ailments such as diabetes, heart disease, blood pressure or cholesterol, YOU DO HAVE A WAY OUT. Why wouldn't you want to get well and have a natural lifespan, complication-free? Choosing inaction means choosing a premature end to your life. The question is, "What choice will you make?"

Proper Blood Pressure Monitoring Technique And Frequency of Measurement

Here Follows the Story of Tyrone, Who Monitors His Blood Pressure ONLY at Every Doctor Visit, and the Danger That Created for Him

"Janet, in-between doctor visits, 3 to 6 months may lapse; and during this period, if you don't monitor on a daily basis, your blood pressure may skyrocket and cause a major stroke or a heart attack, without warning. Your life, as you know it, may be shattered in a flash. You can avoid these strokes and heart attacks by diligently monitoring your blood pressure, and when it starts climbing above 130/80, and then you will alert your doctor to rectify it. I see this problem occurring every day, in my practice. Out of every 10 people I counsel, maybe one or two monitor on a regular basis, take their medications consistently, remain active and make good food choices. The remaining 80% either don't take blood pressure medications as prescribed, don't monitor periodically on a daily basis, remain sedentary all day long, and eat and drink without limits; these are the ones who, consequently, are paying the ultimate price." That is why I keep repeating to you and every one else those important messages about monitoring and lifestyle changes because the majority of people do not pay attention to them and they miss out.

My pharmacist colleagues, all over the nation, and I encounter these same, unfortunate, and totally preventable situations; we see them repeated **every day**, repeated by **MILLIONS of people** with chronic conditions. Just yesterday, Janet, a middle-aged guy named Tyrone, who couldn't be more than about 54 years old, came into the pharmacy. He was a bit overweight and was a smoker. He came up to the counter and asked me about over-the-counter medications for congestion. The first thing I asked was whether he took blood pressure medication; he replied, "Yes." When I asked how often he monitors his blood pressure and how much his last reading was, he replied that he does not monitor on his own. He waits for the doctor to take it at his office, and he goes to the doctor about twice a year. So that's once every 6 months that he monitors his blood pressure. His last blood pressure reading was 160/95. He replied that his doctor increased his medication a while back, but he did not know what his reading currently was.

I suggested he take a reading at the free blood pressure machine at the pharmacy corner and instructed him on the proper measuring procedure. To our surprise, Tyrone's reading was 165/105 (a walking time bomb) with a pulse of 87 (the average resting pulse is 70). A higher pulse rate indicates a less fit heart due to a sedentary lifestyle. He admitted to me, that since his last doctor's visit, he had been watching a lot more TV at the start of the football season while snacking on enormous amounts of chips, popcorn and all kind of "goodies" and washing all these down with several cans of beer or regular soft drinks daily or several times a week. He also said that he thought he did not need to take his blood pressure medication every day; but mostly, he has been taking his pills "a couple times a week," or "when I feel I really need them." In addition, he admitted to gaining about 15 pounds since his last doctor's visit.

I strongly advised Tyrone to take his medications on a regular basis, to monitor his blood pressure daily or at least 5 times per week and keep a log of his readings, and to aim at a blood pressure level of below 130/80. I also recommended some lifestyle changes addressing the consumption of enormous amounts of booze and food and his sedentary lifestyle. I also strongly urged him to contact his doctor immediately, to inform him of his current blood pressure reading in order to rectify the problem as soon as possible and avoid a possible heart attack or a stroke. The pressure in his head may have been due, not only to his sinuses, but to elevated blood pressure levels. For his sinus complaint, I suggested he only take Tylenol or Ibuprofen for the pain, and also suggested he use nasal saline spray to keep his sinuses flushed and moist, which reduces sinus discomfort and pressure; I also instructed him to use a vaporizer. Most importantly, I recommended he take his blood pressure medications as prescribed and that he monitor his pressure daily. I also urged lifestyle changes by making better snacking and food choices and substituting some TV watching time with some walking and moving around activity.

Here Follows the Story of Ricardo, Who Had a Near-Stroke-Level Blood Pressure Reading and Was Near Collapse

In another instance, Janet, a Hispanic fellow named Ricardo, who was also middle-aged, showed up to the pharmacy-counseling window, wanting advice. I could tell, by his demeanor, that he was distraught and not feeling very well. He asked me what he could take for his pounding headache. The first question I asked him was about his blood pressure and whether he was on any medication. He replied that he was a diabetic and that he did have blood pressure problems, but he said he was no longer taking his medications. At that point, my heart started pulsing with worry. When I inquired further, it turned out that he could not afford the medications the doctor had prescribed him, and added that he'd stopped taking his medications about a month prior. When I asked him about his last blood pressure reading, he replied that it had probably been several months since he'd had a reading taken.

I asked him to sit at the blood pressure monitor, right there, at the pharmacy, for a couple of minutes, in order to have him rest and to take a reading for me. He literally dragged himself the few steps it took to get to the machine, and he seemed to be further distraught. When he completed the reading, his blood pressure was 170/110. I immediately suggested he go to the emergency room and better yet, I proposed that we call 911 for him and seek immediate medical treatment. Having out of control diabetes, combined with high cholesterol and very high blood pressure, is a formula for an imminent heart attack or a major stroke; I anticipated this final outcome, in the back of my mind; and I was not about to let that happen on my clock. He adamantly refused the idea; he said he was okay and that he was going to resume taking his blood pressure medication, repeating, "everything will be fine." But I knew better; I insisted and was not about to let him walk away in this shape.

He continued refusing my suggestion, and he just walked away from the counseling window. Although I cannot force people to do something they don't want to do, I felt in my heart that he was going to be in trouble if I did not take action and fast. I followed him to the exit door, and I saw him sitting on the bench right before the exit door, trying to catch his breath. When I approached him, he readily agreed to get help. I suggested he remain there until the emergency personnel arrived. My technician had already called 911, and after only few minutes the emergency crew was on the scene. They immediately measured his blood pressure; it had already shot up to 180/120. The paramedics rushed him to the hospital. I found out, as I had suspected, that he had high cholesterol, as well, and that he had stopped taking his medications for cholesterol as well.

Ricardo was on a suicide mission without knowing it. Several days later, a healthier-looking Ricardo showed up to the counter, and with a genuine smile, he shook my hand and thanked me for "saving his life." The doctor at that hospital told him that had he waited much longer, he would have certainly had a major stroke, a heart attack or worse. He got back on a bunch of medications to control all of his problems; but since he was on a budget, his doctor prescribed medications that were available in an equally effective, but much cheaper generic form that he can afford. He learned his lesson, he said; and he promised me that he would take his medications as prescribed, and that he would start monitoring his blood pressure and sugar as I suggested.

Selecting a Blood Pressure Monitor and Cuff Size

I think these stories I told Janet hit the right note with her. Janet rushed back to tell me she was convinced that daily blood pressure monitoring was important and said that she wanted to start monitoring her own blood pressure daily. Janet proceeded to ask me,

"Which blood pressure machine should I buy?"
"What is a good choice without breaking my budget?"

I replied, "Janet, blood pressure machines are available from the fully manual to the fully automated, which can give you printouts." The price varies from the fully manual at about $19 to the fully automated at about $120 or more. They all have almost the same accuracy, but it is just a matter of choosing how automated you want it and deciding what features you want and can afford.

I recommended a machine that takes only one push to activate and which requires the least task-coordination. You really do not need the more expensive ones that give you a printout. You place the cuff in the right direction on your left arm (proper blood pressure measuring procedure is provided a couple paragraphs down), and then you push one button; within seconds the machine inflates, deflates, and gives you a reading that can be stored in the machine's memory. These machines are usually the most economical. Wal-Mart has its own brand of these blood pressure machines. They cost about $45, and they are manufactured for them by a brand-company by the name of Omron. Omron is a very reputable company that manufactures a wide range of health-related products and monitors.

Always select the arm monitors instead of the wrist or the finger monitors. The arm monitor is the most accurate. If, for some reason, an arm monitor cannot be used, then a wrist monitor may be an alternative. Omron puts out a wrist monitor that uses satellite positioning and may be more accurate than other wrist monitors. But never rely on the finger monitors. They're not accurate.

Most retail pharmacies have their own FREE sit-in blood pressure monitors. If you don't own a monitor and want to monitor your blood pressure with these machines, always choose the same machine. It is not accurate to go measure your blood pressure with several machines STICK WITH THE SAME MACHINE for maximum accuracy. And remember, keep a written log, as a back up to the memory, of these readings to take to and share with your doctor. If your blood pressure starts climbing above 130/80, call your doctor immediately, DO NOT WAIT for your next visit.

Proper Cuff Size

The arm monitors that are sold in stores, and the stationary sit-in blood pressure monitors that you find at your local drug stores, are designed for people with average arm sizes. Consequently, if someone has a thin or a larger arm size, then these monitors will not provide accurate readings and should not be used. If the arm fits snuggly in the blood pressure machine, the reading should not proceed. Likewise, if the arm fits loosely then again you should not proceed. There are large and small cuff-sizes that are sold separately; they come in an assortment of sizes. You can find them at retail pharmacies and pharmacies that specialize in selling medical supplies. Just make sure that the cuff-size brand you choose fits the monitor you are buying. Also, the manufacturers of these blood pressure monitors "can be contacted," and you can order large or small cuff-sizes directly through them that will be a match for your monitor.

How to Get an Accurate Blood Pressure-Reading

Janet, I suggest you monitor your blood pressure daily if possible, or at least 4-5 times a week. The best time to take your blood pressure is first thing in the morning before you had coffee, tea, or any caffeinated beverage or tobacco products or 45 minutes after consuming such products; otherwise you can get a false reading. If you are a smoker, I urge you to quit as soon as possible, as recommended by my smoking cessation guide "Stop Smoking Today." Take the blood pressure reading in your left arm since it is closer to your heart and the reading is slightly more accurate, unless for various reasons you are not able to do so. If, for some reason, you cannot take the blood pressure reading using the left arm, then right arm reading is okay.

Home Blood Pressure-Monitoring Technique

Before taking your reading, you should have been sitting and relaxing for about five minutes. Your arm should be at heart level, resting on a pillow or a table. Your body and posture must be upright and relaxed, and your legs should be straight and not crossed while sitting. Breathe normally, relax, and do not talk until the procedure is completed. If any of the above criteria have been breached, then you must start again. Slide the cuff on your arm so that it reaches slightly above your elbow, and position it in the way it's recommended by your monitor. Generally, most cuffs have a sign indicating the proper positioning of that cuff. Read your instruction manual carefully before using that blood pressure monitor. Then press the start button and stay put for the ride.

The cuff will self-inflate then deflate slowly; right towards the end of complete deflation, you will get some numbers displayed on your screen. You will get a higher reading, which is your systolic blood pressure reading (the pressure when your heart is in action), and then you will get a lower reading, which is your diastolic blood pressure reading (the pressure when your heart is in a very brief rest period), and a pulse reading. Although most monitors have memories, I still suggest you write the results down in your blood pressure notebook; your entries should each include the date and time. It is a good idea to keep that log, because it comes in handy when you go to the doctor's office and want to show them your readings. (You're able to track any steady rise above 130/80 when you have several readings in your pocket notebook).

BLOOD PRESSURE-MONITORING TECHNIQUE IN THE PHARMACY

Most pharmacies now have "free" blood pressure-monitoring machines where you can sit and take your reading. Some machines are more sophisticated than others, as they can also measure your weight and BMI. Here are some tips to help you get more accurate readings and avoid false high readings, as I have been witnessing in pharmacies all throughout my practice. I see people rush to the blood pressure machine as they just finished a cup of coffee or put down their cigarette, and this, possibly combined with over-the-counter sinus medications which can transiently raise their blood pressure and provide a false reading. Ideally, you need to sit at the machine for about 4 or 5 minutes before pushing the start button. Relax, breathe normally, and keep your legs straight, and do not talk while the reading is in progress. Then slide your arm in the cuff until it's slightly above the elbow, and then press the start button.

When the measurement is in progress, keep breathing normally and don't converse with anybody, even if we call you into the pharmacy to tell you that your prescription is ready.

Regarding clothing, if you're wearing a very thin shirt, it may be okay to take the reading with the shirtsleeve in place. However, anything thicker, such as a sweater, will provide a false reading. Slide your shirt up, and make sure it doesn't squeeze your arm too much when it's up, because then again, it can give you a false reading. How many times should you repeat the test each time? I have seen people test every 3 minutes in order to get a lower reading. It doesn't work that way. The maximum you can try is twice, and within 5 or 10 minutes of each other. If you do it more, then the blood will be engorged in your arm, and it's going to give you a false reading, again.

I then asked Janet, since she was right there at the pharmacy, and since we had a blood pressure machine at our disposal, to take a blood pressure reading. So Janet followed the appropriate blood pressure measurement technique: she sat at the machine for a few minutes, and then she took a reading. Her pressure came out to be 142/89 with a pulse of 84. This reading was consistent with that of the doctor's, which was 140/90. "What is the magic blood pressure target?" I asked Janet. She replied, "Below 130/80. My blood pressure is elevated."

WHAT IS A NORMAL RESTING PULSE?

Janet inquired about her resting pulse being 84 and wondered what a normal resting pulse reading should be. I told Janet that an average resting pulse is about 70 beats per minute. A higher resting pulse rate in the absence of any heart condition is an indication that she may be leading a sedentary lifestyle and that her heart is not "fit." I also explained that her heart, which is a very complex muscle, has to do more work. When Janet becomes more fit, her resting pulse will start dropping slowly to about 70 or less beats per minute. I told Janet, that as we grow older and we become more sedentary; this not only puts more and more strain and wear on our heart, but I reminded her that a sedentary lifestyle begets weight gain, which places further strain on the heart. Soon, heart problems become inevitable, and it is only a matter of time before that sedentary individual who has a weight problem could have a sudden heart attack or a stroke. I also suggested to Janet to refer to the lifestyle section in this guide to have a better understanding of how she can begin implementing an active lifestyle and make more balanced food choices, at the same time, losing weight (without having to engage in fad or crash diets) and permanently maintaining that weight loss.

I then asked Janet to hand me the prescription that her doctor had given her for her blood pressure, so that we could get it filled and get her started on it in order to begin reducing her blood pressure and get it at the desired level, below 130/80. After her prescription was completed, I requested that she come back to the window so I could explain more about her blood pressure medication.

"Janet, let me explain to you a little bit about your blood pressure medication that you will be taking, *and the other classes of blood pressure lowering medications which we will discuss in this upcoming section.* However, before I start, I want to remind you that the only reason I'm giving you the explanation about these drugs is not for you or anyone else taking these medications to become experts or to make personal decisions about treatment without consulting with the doctor, but for you and others to be involved in your own treatment by understanding the necessity of taking them regularly and reporting, to your doctor or pharmacist, anything that is "not right." It's very important to keep taking the medication as prescribe and not take any actions regarding your treatment before consulting with your doctor; and if you have any inquiries, you can also consult with your pharmacist. (Please refer to the beginning of Action Step 2, where I provide, in detail, the dangers of people making personal decisions about their treatment before consulting with their pharmacist or doctor).

NOTE: This upcoming discussion is for the curious only. You may read valuable and simple information about the drugs you are currently taking for blood pressure. You may also read about them at a later stage. Otherwise, you can forward to the next and crucially important section Action Step 4.

The Several Classes of Blood Pressure Medications that Are Ideal For People Who Have Diabetes

"Janet, there are several classes of blood pressure medications, each working in a different manner to lower your blood pressure. It is not uncommon for your doctor to put you on several of them, each belonging to a different class that lowers your blood pressure in different ways, in order to reach the target blood pressure of below 130/80. Since you are diabetic, there are some classes of blood pressure medication that would be ideal for you. The prescription that your doctor prescribed, Lisinopril/HCTZ 20/12.5, belongs to a line of blood pressure lowering medications called ACE inhibitors for people like you, who have diabetes.

ACE Inhibitors not only lower your blood pressure but also protect and prevent your heart, kidneys, and blood vessels from further problems and damage. The other component of the drug your doctor prescribed is HCTZ, which stands for "Hydrochlorothiazide" (you do not have to remember that long word), which is a water pill. Water pills help rid your body from excess fluid, reducing the volume of water in your blood vessels, consequently reducing your blood pressure in the process. More details on this group of medications will be discussed a little later in this guide.

ACE Inhibitors
How Do They Work?

ACE inhibitors stand for Angiotensin Converting Enzyme Inhibitors, which exert their blood pressure-lowering effect by preventing the formation of a blood pressure-raising substance in the kidneys called Angiotensin.

Older drugs belonging to this class, alone or in combination with diuretics are taken 2 to 3 times daily and they are:

- Vasotec(generic: Enalapril)
- Vaseretic (generic: Enalapril + HCTZ)
- Capoten (generic: Captopril)
- Capozide(generic: Captropril + HCTZ)

The newer medications in this class requiring more convenient once or twice daily dosing are, in random order:

- Accupril (generic: Quinapril)
- Accuzide (generic: Quinapril + HCTZ)
- Lotensin (generic: Benazepril)
- Lotensin HCT (generic: Benazepril + HCTZ)
- Zestril or Prinivil (generic: Lisinopril)
- Zestoretic or Prinizide (generic: Lisinpril + HCTZ)
- Univasc (generic: Moxapril)
- Uniretic (generic: Moxapril + HCTZ)
- Monopril (generic :Fosinopril)
- Monopril HCT (generic: Fosinopril + HCTZ)

All of the above are available in much less expensive equally effective generic brands, and I highly recommend always choosing generics on any drug that's available. They are equally effective as the brand, but at a much lesser cost, which makes it more affordable to treat your condition.

The following are only available in brand names, but generics are coming out soon:

- Altace (Ramipril)
- Aceon (Perindopril)
- Mavik (Trandolapril)

There is available a frequently-used blood pressure lowering drug combining the convenience and the potential effects of two aggressive groups of blood pressure-lowering drugs. The drug is called:

- Lotrel (Benazepril and Norvasc): Benazepril belongs to the ACE Inhibitors family and Norvasc belongs to what is called Calcium Channel Blockers.

Each drug lowers blood pressure in a different manner and the combination of their effects in one convenient pill is relatively unique and worth mentioning.

What Dose Is Right for Me?

Your doctor, Janet, will determine the dose that is suitable for you and others. You just take it as prescribed every day. Generally, your doctor should start you on the lowest effective dose and work his or her way up according to your blood pressure response in order to reach an end target of keeping your blood pressure, most of the time, below the magic number of 130/80.

Your doctor should reassess your treatment in 3 to 4 weeks after he/she starts you on any new medications for blood pressure, because it takes that long before you can see the maximum benefit with that new treatment. However, unless your blood pressure is very high, say over 160/95 or 170/100, then your doctor needs to take initial aggressive measures to quickly lower your blood pressure to a safer zone.

What Should I Know about the Side Effects of ACE Inhibitors?

Well, Janet, first off, before we start talking about side effects, it is important for you to know that any side effect that might occur does NOT occur 100% of the time or in all people. These side effects occur in much smaller percentages anywhere from .5% to 1% (or sometimes slightly higher percentages), and again, they may or may not occur. And that applies to all medications. ACE Inhibitors are a group of medications that are well tolerated, but you might experience the following:

1. With the first few doses, you might experience some drowsiness. To resolve the situation, if it occurs, take the medications initially at night, before bedtime. And after a few days, you can switch to the morning dose. This lightheadedness with the first few doses is a common occurrence and may be transient. That's one of the reasons your doctor starts you on the lowest effective dose, initially.

2. Persistent dry cough. It is important for you to know, Janet, that if you develop a persistent cough at any time while on any ACE Inhibitor treatment, let your doctor know; and the cough should resolve when the drug is changed either to another ACE Inhibitor or to another class of medications. ACE Inhibitors are known to cause this mild and reversible nuisance of persistent dry cough.

**Potential Side Effects Requiring Your Full Attention
And Your Doctor's Intervention:**

1. *A rise in potassium levels*: ACE inhibitors may cause a rise in potassium levels, and this problem can be compounded when taken with other medications that also cause that same effect in the blood. Such medications are potassium supplements (either prescription or over-the-counter), and water pills that have the ability to hold potassium in your body, such as Maxide (HCTZ + Triamterene), Dyazide (HCTZ + Triamterene in a capsule form), Aldactone (Spironolactone), and the most recent, Inspra (Eplerenone). Also salt substitutes containing potassium salts can be an additional potential problem in raising potassium levels in your blood. Bananas, oranges, and orange juice are all rich sources of potassium. Take special care when consuming these fruits along with the other problem drugs and supplements we just discussed that could raise potassium. Balanced potassium levels in your body cells and blood are crucial for regular heartbeats. Potassium levels that are out of whack can cause heart problems and, ultimately, can be life threatening if not addressed promptly.

    <u>Solution:</u>

    - Remind your doctor of frequent blood potassium level checks, especially when taking other potassium-raising drugs and potassium supplements, as discussed.
    - Do not consume salt substitutes containing potassium.

2. Another major, rare and reversible side effect is fluid build-up around your facial and breathing areas, causing these areas to swell up, making it difficult for you to breathe.

    <u>Solution:</u>

    - Although this reaction is rare, at the first sign of lip, tongue, mouth or throat-swelling, or at the first sign of difficulty swallowing or breathing, stop the medication immediately and have someone take you to the nearest emergency room or call emergency services at 911. Again, this is a reversible situation. This condition is referred to in technical terms as Angioedema (you don't have to remember this term). African Americans are more vulnerable to this problem than other ethnic groups.

Who Should NOT Take This Group of Medications?

If you are pregnant, planning to become pregnant or nursing, do not take this line of blood pressure medications, as they can cause harm to your baby.

What Other Drugs Interact with ACE Inhibitors?

Generally, this group of drugs has a low occurrence of drug interactions:

1. Drugs that are referred to as "NSAID," such as Ibuprofen, Naprosyn (Aleve, Naproxen, and Anaprox), Indomethacin (Indocin), Celebrex, Mobic, and others may slightly reduce the effect of the ACE Inhibitor group. As you regularly monitor your blood pressure, you need to inform your doctor of any fluctuations in your blood pressure.

2. Take antacids such as Maalox, Mylanta, PeptoBismol, Rolaids and Tums, about 2 hours apart from any other medications you are taking, including ACE Inhibitors.

What Your Doctor Should Be Monitoring Periodically:

- Your kidney functions, as the ACE inhibitor drugs are eliminated by your kidneys.
- Your potassium levels (as discussed previously).

"Janet, just remember that all adverse situations occur in a very small number of people, and when they do occur, they are manageable and reversible. This is an excellent line of blood pressure-lowering medications, and their benefits to you and others who take any medication from this line far outweighs any adverse situation that is manageable and that "might" occur. Now that you have become better informed, you will know what to expect and what to do if any situation comes up."

Janet seemed to be intrigued by the ACE inhibitor story; "Those are simple and very important tips you have just given me about my medications. You had mentioned that there are other groups of blood pressure-lowering medications that are ideal for me as a diabetic, namely, the water pill component in the medication my doctor prescribed.

So How Do Water Pills Work and Why Are They an Important Addition to My Treatment?

There are many kinds of water pills, but HCTZ (you do not need to remember the full name which is Hydrochlorothiazide) is the one used first line for people who have diabetes, and that is the one I will tell you about since the other fluid pills may lower the effect of the ACE Inhibitors or interact with them.

These fluid pills work by ridding the body, through the kidneys, of excess salt, which is referred to as sodium. When sodium leaves the body through the urine, water is automatically lost and follows the sodium, leaving the body through the urine as well. Consequently, the fluid amount in the blood is reduced, which creates less pressure on the arteries, eventually reducing the overall pressure in this fashion.

African Americans who have high blood pressure are more vulnerable to the effects of blood pressure lowering of these fluid pills than other ethnic groups. Fluid pills are integral for lowering blood pressure, especially for African Americans.

What Side Effects Could These Fluid Pills Have?

The benefits of any treatment are weighed against the consequences. Any side effects I will tell you about happen to a small percentage of people, and they are manageable. Definitely, the benefits of fluid pills far outweigh any consequences. Some of the side effects are or could be:

- Drowsiness with the first few doses (will tend to go away)
- An increase in uric acid: a rise in uric acid is possible when taking HTCZ; this may cause a flare up of gout. Therefore, people who have gout need to have their uric acid checked periodically at the doctor's office.
- Increase in sugar levels: A rise in sugar levels is also possible when taking these fluid pills. Since you are now monitoring your sugar daily, as we have discussed earlier, then you will notice a rise, if any, when taking HCTZ fluid pill. Nowadays, lower dosages such as 12.5 mg are recommended over higher ones, which would still be effective in lowering your blood pressure but present a lesser chance of side effects. Higher HCTZ doses are more effective but will cause more side effects. Your doctor will make decisions based on benefits vs. consequences.
- Increase in cholesterol levels: You're going to be surprised about this side effect. HCTZ **may** cause a small rise in cholesterol levels. You might rush to the conclusion and say, "Well then, I am going to stop this medication right now." Now hold on to your horses. You should not rush to any conclusion or action before consulting with your pharmacist or doctor. You do not have the full background to make such a decision. The doctor should be monitoring your cholesterol levels anyway; any rise in your cholesterol will show in the lab results, and your doctor will resolve this situation to your benefit. Problem solved.
- Decrease in potassium levels: HCTZ may cause a decline in potassium levels. If you consume potassium-rich foods like banana and oranges then

your potassium levels may be okay. Your doctor may elect to put you on potassium supplements, depending on your potassium levels, in order to offset that potassium loss. Since Lisinopril, which belongs to the ACE Inhibitors group, may cause a rise in potassium levels this rise can be offset by the loss of potassium HCTZ can cause.

Other Matters to Be Concerned with while Taking the Fluid Pill:

- Avoid prolonged sun exposure, since HCTZ may make your skin more sensitive to the effects of sun, and you may burn more easily. You may need to apply a sun block of SPF 30 on the exposed parts of your skin. Applying a sun block is not a protection against drugs that sensitize your skin for sun problems. The best thing to do is to avoid sun exposure by wearing a hat, staying in the shade, and wearing long-sleeved loose-fitting clothing.
- *Sulfa allergies*: Another possible problem you need to be aware of is that if you are allergic to Sulfa drugs, you may be allergic to HCTZ. But it's not a given. Be on the lookout for any rash on your skin or itching which usually happens at the start of the treatment. If a rash develops, stop the medication immediately and contact your doctor, and start taking Benadryl (over-the-counter - which is 25 mg), and if you are an adult, take 2 capsules every 6 hours, which is 4 times a day, for the next 2-3 days. Beware that Benadryl may cause drowsiness.

What Other Groups of Blood Pressure Medications Are Ideal for People with Diabetes?

There is a very important group of drugs called Angiotensin Receptor Blockers referred to as ARBs, related to the ACE Inhibitors, which are just as beneficial; not only are they very effective blood pressure-lowering drugs, but they also protect your heart and kidneys from the damage of disease progression. They act as a shield to your heart and kidneys, like ACE but are slightly more aggressive in that protective effect and in lowering blood pressure and preventing heart complications. ARBs work almost like ACE Inhibitors in lowering your blood pressure. All side effects, drug interactions, and various factors that we have discussed for ACE Inhibitors are the same for ACE Blockers. With regard to the persistent cough nuisance, the ARBs have less of an occurrence. Your doctor will determine the appropriate dose of any medications for you.

Drugs in the ARB group in random order are:

- Cozaar
- Hyzaar (Cozaar plus HCTZ)
- Diovan
- Diovan HCT
- Avapro
- Avalide (Avapro plus HCTZ)
- Atacand HCT
- Atacand
- Micardis
- Micardis HCT
- Teveten
- Teveten HCT

The HCT additional component is the same as with the ACE inhibitors group and is referred to as HCTZ, which is the water pill. None of these drugs are available in generic form yet, since they are relatively more recent than the ACE Inhibitor group.

Who Is a Favorite Candidate for These ARB Drugs?

If someone who has diabetes has the start of kidney damage, which is a condition called Micro Albuminuria, or in other words, loss of some form of protein in the urine, which is a step before total kidney failure then the ARBs are used first line to protect the kidneys from further damage. **It is paramount to mention that, at this stage of the start of kidney failure, total kidney failure can be prevented by reducing blood pressure, sugar levels, and cholesterol levels aggressively and by adopting favorable lifestyle habits and losing even a small amount of weight.**

Others with blood pressure problems will benefit tremendously from these medications. If you do not have medical insurance, and since these are not yet available in generic form and can be pricey, then the generic drugs in the ACE Inhibitors group are a great alternative.

What Should the Doctor Monitor Periodically When I Am on ACE Blockers?

Just like the ACE Inhibitors group, monitoring kidney function and potassium level is paramount.

The Last Group of Potential Blood Pressure Lowering Drugs That We Will Discuss Is Beta Blockers

Beta Blockers are one more very powerful group of blood pressure-lowering medications, which are ideal for people with diabetes; they are not only aggressive in lowering blood pressure but are also protective to your heart. Out of all other groups of blood pressure-lowering medication, Beta Blockers are unique in their heart protective properties. If a person with diabetes has already had a heart attack, then Beta Blockers alone or in combination with ACE Inhibitors or ACE Blockers, with or without a water pill, are ideally prescribed. Janet asked me, "I have heard of Beta Blockers before, but why are they called that and how do they work?"

How Beta Blockers Work and Ideal Candidates

Janet, this class of blood pressure medication works by blocking what is called the Beta receptors in the blood vessels and in your heart, and consequently prevent some blood pressure-raising nerve substances from binding to these receptors and causing your blood pressure to rise. The result is not only a blood pressure-lowering effect, but Beta Blockers reduce your heart rate at rest and during exercise, making your heart work more efficiently and with less effort. This makes this class of drugs very effective for people who have had a heart attack or heart failure.

What Medications Fall into This Category?

For people with Diabetes, the preferred drugs in this category are in random order:

- Lopressor (Metoprolol)
- Lopressor HCTZ (Metoprolol + HCTZ)
- Tenormin (Atenolol)
- Tenoretic (Atenolol + HCTZ)
- Ziac (bisoprolol + HCTZ)
- Bisoprolol

All these drugs are available in generic form; and again, I recommend selecting generic drugs when available. **Toprol XL** is the same as Lopressor but in a sustained release form (not yet available in a generic form but will be soon).

Although there are many other drugs in the Beta Blocker family, these are the most widely prescribed because they create the least problems regarding breathing and do not affect the blood sugar levels like the other members of the Beta Blocker family.

Your doctor will make a decision about which drug is best for you and which dose is appropriate.

What Common Side Effects Can Beta Blockers Cause?

While on any of these medications, you can expect:

- Dizziness.
- Stomach problems, either diarrhea or constipation.
- **Fatigue** (this can occur at any time while on Beta Blockers and can start several months after you have been on any of them. Then again, a small percentage of people may develop this nuisance, and changing the medication or changing the class of drugs can remedy it. So if you are on Beta Blocker medication/s and you start noticing that you are **tired** all of the time, it is likely that the Beta Blocker is what's causing that problem).
- Hypotension (a drop in blood pressure).

A Common Problem that Can Occur with Beta Blockers And with Most Blood Pressure Medications

Orthostatic Hypotension is a sudden drop in your blood pressure after you stand up or, for instance, if you bend down to pick something up from the floor and try to stand up again, you feel that you become light-headed (some people may pass out); this is due to a sudden drop in blood pressure.

To avoid this sudden drop in blood pressure, if you are getting out of bed, sit on the edge of the bed for a few seconds and then stand very slowly. The same applies if you've been sitting at the dining table and want to stand (whenever you move from any seated position to a standing position, try to move to a standing position very slowly). If the phone rings, do not rush from your seated position to try to pick up the phone, don't rush your movement after sitting, for any reason, as you might get light-headed and pass out on your way down a flight of stairs and bump your head somewhere. The problem is graver if you are taking blood-thinning medication such as Aspirin, Coumadin Plavix, Ticlid, Persantine and Aggrenox, and you fall and hit your head then internal bleeding in your brain can occur and the consequences are dire. To resolve this situation, just stand very slowly, and that problem will be minimized.

What Other Very Important Information Should I Know about Beta Blockers?

- It is best to take these medications with food, since the nature of some of these medications favors a fatty medium; consequently, their absorption is improved when consumed with a meal that has moderate fat content.

- Do not make decisions on your own about increasing or decreasing the dose of any medication, including this one. If, accidentally, you miss a one-day dose of any blood pressure medication, especially these, then continue with the next scheduled dose. Do not double up on your medication the next day.
- **Beta Blockers should not be stopped abruptly, as it might cause a sudden heart attack and may cause a sudden rise in blood pressure. If your doctor makes the decision for you to stop this medication, then he or she would have to wean you off of it gradually.**
- Keep physical activity at a minimum if your doctor plans to get you to stop this medication.
- Since Beta Blockers reduce your resting and exercise heart rate, then during a scheduled activity (in other words, exercise) do not monitor your intensity by your pulse rate. Use what is called "the talk test" instead. During exercise, try to gauge your intensity by trying to say a few words. If you are gasping for air after a couple of words, then the intensity is too high; you should slow down a little or drop your arm movement. On the other hand, if while you are walking you are able to say a full couple of sentences before needing to breathe in then this an indication that you are going too slow and you need to pick up your speed and/or add arm motion. You should be able to say 3 or 4 words comfortably before you have to breathe in.

There are several other categories of drugs that are used to treat blood pressure, but they are not all favorable for people who have diabetes; consequently, they will not be discussed here. If you, for any reason, cannot tolerate any of the first line drugs, then your doctor will choose blood pressure drugs from other categories, and there are plenty of them.

Summary of the Various Blood Pressure Drugs And Their Usage

Your doctor will make the right decision as to which drugs or combination of drugs and dosages are right for you. However, to have an idea of how your doctor might select one over the other, for instance, I will share the following:

For people who have diabetes and blood pressure but have no kidney or heart problems, your doctor might elect to choose a first line drug treatment from either the ACE Inhibitors or the ARB Group, and possibly add a water pill if your blood pressure is not coming down to below 130/80.

If your doctor suspects the beginning of kidney problems, then again ACE Inhibitors or ARBs are ideal as first line. If somebody has kidney failure or kidney damage, then ARBs are definitely used as first line.

If somebody with diabetes has already had a heart attack, then Beta Blockers become first choice with or without the use of ACE Inhibitors, ARBs and water pills, but water pills are typically prescribed.

"Janet, I hope I was able to give you a better understanding of all the various issues related to your condition. I urge you, and I wish from the bottom of my heart that you would start acting on the information I gave you; if you do, you will literally transform your life and reclaim control of your health, and you will move away from the daily threats of complications due to diabetes." I told Janet that I have to go back to filling prescriptions, as I was getting very backed up. Janet looked me in the eyes, extended her hand, shook mine and genuinely thanked me. She also promised me that she would start acting on the advice I gave her.

WHAT YOU ABSOLUTELY MUST KNOW AT A GLANCE FROM ACTION STEP 3

The third and crucial step in deciphering the "magic formula" for "ultimate diabetes control" and peace of mind:

TAKE ACTION NOW:

- Start monitoring your sugar, cholesterol, blood pressure and other vital parameters as recommended in the MAGIC COMPASS TABLE that every diabetic can not afford to live without in order to avoid the deadly complications of diabetes (Page 72).

- Lower your cholesterol to the "under control" magic numbers that are revealed to you on Page 72 and make use of the various drugs available to treat cholesterol and make sure you know all you should know about them in order to avoid an earth-shattering heart attack and stroke (starting on Page 79).

- Lower your blood pressure to the magic "under control" numbers and avoid a major life changing heart attack, stroke or kidney failure and find out about the various drugs available to help you successfully lower your blood pressure (starting on Page 90).

Action Step 4:
Lifestyle Choices

Learn to Make Favorable Lifestyle Choices; Learn How to Build New Good Habits; Make Favorable Food and Activity Choices; Lose Weight Permanently without Ever Dieting Again

Our lives and health are precious miracles, and we must take an active and leading role in preserving these divine and physical gifts. Adults are role models to kids. Informed adults who have diabetes and who make wiser meal and snack choices, who also shift gradually to a more active lifestyle and involve all the family in these choices, will reap the rewards; not only for themselves, but those rewards will reach to all family members, including any overweight children who will learn from these parents' actions. The plusses of parents who make conscious favorable food and activity choices are endless. It's a positive for the adults and their children.

FAVORABLE LIFESTYLE CHOICES

The Rewards to You, the Diabetic, If You Continue to Persistently Make Favorable Lifestyle Choices

- Your body will respond optimally to the effects of medications.
- Your blood sugar levels and blood pressure will be "under control" and much closer to the recommended levels in "the magic compass table" on page 72.
- Your bad cholesterol and triglycerides will decline, and your good cholesterol will increase.
- Your risk for heart disease will be drastically reduced.

- You will be able to lose weight and maintain that loss permanently; and by doing so, you will lower your chances of ever having chronic diseases.
- You will enjoy a more zealous quality of life and expect to achieve a natural lifespan.
- Your **sexual health** will improve dramatically.
- You will have positively influenced those around you and those who look up to you, such as your children.
- **You will save money** in the short and long run, because the risk of treating complications is reduced. If all possible complications are reduced or eliminated, you will need fewer medications, and even your current medications/dosages may be reduced. You will be spending more time enjoying your life with your loved ones instead of spending that time in the hospital recovering from avoidable complications.

Starting the change towards a healthier lifestyle is going to be at the heart of your quest to achieve and maintain good health and to be able to avert all the debilitating and life-threatening diabetes complications; you will consequently be able to enjoy the ultimate quality of life. **By lifestyle changes, I mean establishing and maintaining new and favorable habits of** *choosing* **to:**

- Consume balanced meals
- Increase your daily activity levels
- Reduce your stress levels

And if you are a smoker, consider quitting smoking as soon as possible by referring to my guide "Stop Smoking Today."

But you say, "It's easier said than done." And you might ask:

- What are the components of a balanced meal for me, as somebody who has diabetes?
- Will I be deprived of sweets for the rest of my life?
- Do I have to lose a lot of weight to get my diabetes and blood pressure under control?
- And how do I lose weight?
- How much activity do I have to do?
- Do I have to go to the gym and work out for 2 hours every day before I can see noticeable results?
- What activities are good for me and for how long do I do them?
- How do I start and maintain these habits?

- How do I incorporate all of this in my busy day?
- How can I quit smoking for good? (The process of quitting smoking will not be discussed in this guide. My smoking cessation guide " Stop Smoking Today" will help you quit for good. Check the end of this guide for my contact information and website for information on how to purchase this guide.)

That's what we will be discussing next.

The Story of Wanda's Son Who Is Diabetic and Bakes Cookies And Eats Them in Large Quantities:

A few months ago, I was working at a pharmacy in Dallas and I learned that Wanda, one of the technicians I worked with, had diabetes. She was overweight; her blood sugar and cholesterol levels were out of control even though she was taking medications for all of these ailments. Over a period of time, I tried to coach her (as much as my workload at the pharmacy would allow) on various issues such as blood sugar, blood pressure and cholesterol monitoring, appropriate medications and dosages as well as lifestyle matters, such as balanced food intake and activity. She was compliant and eager to improve. One day, she revealed to me that her main concern was her son, who is 33 years old, who also had diabetes; but his diabetes situation was desperate and terribly out of control.

I could really feel her pain and anguish as she was discussing this matter with me. So, I tried to comfort her, and after further probing, I found out that her son weighed 325 pounds, and although he was taking diabetes medications, the last time he took his blood sugar test, it was 298 points; needless to say, his blood pressure and cholesterol were sky high. I was curious and wanted to know more, so I asked her to tell me about his lifestyle, what he'd been eating and how active he was. She then told me that he would sit in front of the TV at least 5-6 hours a day and did nothing but bake cookies and eat them several times a day in massive amounts. She went on to say that she noticed this pattern of snacking on cookies started right around his diagnosis with diabetes a couple years ago. He felt that he did not want to be deprived of sweets and wanted to feel that he was not any different than his friends or other people and made an opposite reaction. It seemed to me that Wanda's son first needed to accept his condition and come to terms with it and realize that he can lead a normal lifestyle and he can eat desserts just like others, but in a balanced fashion; and he must engage in an active lifestyle.

I told Wanda that her son needed to realize that he absolutely could control his diabetes by taking his medications properly, by monitoring his blood glucose, blood pressure and cholesterol levels (as recommended in Section 3 of this guide) and by starting and maintaining favorable lifestyle habits. He needs to gradually increase his level of walking daily and make more balanced food choices to include some of his favorite cookies. He also needed to realize that he was still young and that he has a whole and beautiful life ahead of him, and that he can live a normal lifespan free of any complications, but he must take action immediately and bring his weight and all other parameters down and "under control."

I urged Wanda to relay these messages to her son since he was reluctant to come and talk to me. He needed to know that even if he had diabetes he can still lead a normal life to include desserts and his favorite cookies but in balanced portion sizes and as part of an active and balanced lifestyle.

He also needed to realize that weight loss of as little as 5-7 pounds can make a tremendous improvement in his blood sugar, pressure and cholesterol and his overall diabetes control. His doctor needs to be made aware of his current situation so he can intervene and reevaluate his treatment.

Wanda's son is a classic example of just how important newly diagnosed diabetics need to come to terms with their condition and to realize that diabetes is highly manageable and treatable and very responsive to even small lifestyle changes. Also people with diabetes need to realize that there will not be restrictions to any food including sweets but quantities and portion sizes need to be balanced and moderate and as part of a balanced lifestyle as we will discuss extensively in this Action Step 4. As we will progress into this section you will see that the lifestyle changes and food choices recommendations are the same for diabetics and non-diabetics alike.

Here Is the Story of a Man Who Is Diabetic, Overweight and a Smoker Who "Doesn't Have Time" to Increase His Activity Level!!!

In another instance not long ago, I was working at a retail pharmacy chain in East Texas, and a 50-year-old man with a big belly hanging from his waist, showed up to the pharmacy counter and presented us with seven prescriptions. As he stood there, a glossy cigarette pack was peeking at us from his shirt pocket, and he smelled as if he had just put one out right before he walked into the pharmacy. As my technician was collecting some information from him, I started looking through the scripts. Among others, some of the prescriptions he was getting filled were for his diabetes, high cholesterol and high blood pressure. We told him it was going to be about a 45-minute wait to get the prescriptions filled. He headed to the waiting area and **sat there the entire time!!!**

We got his medications ready. As I was counseling him on the various issues related to the medications, I urged him to consider quitting smoking as soon as possible. When I suggested that he increase his level of activity, guess what he told me. He told me he "doesn't have time" because his work schedule is hectic. This is a common excuse that most people respond with when asked the same question. I hinted to him that he could have been moving around in the store instead of sitting the whole 45 minutes, waiting for his prescriptions. I also indicated to him that both smoking "and" inactivity, separately, contribute in a major way to worsening his diabetes and posing the possibility of all types of life-threatening heart and lung problems. But when smoking, inactivity, obesity and diabetes are combined, then chances of having any kind of fatal complication increases many, many folds.

I urged him to be aware of all these factors and that it takes only minimal effort on his part to start building positive health habits: making wiser food selections from a myriad of food choices that are high in fiber and low in sugar and bad fats; increasing his daily activity at work, at home and while shopping; monitoring his sugar and blood pressure, as I have mentioned for the hundredth time; and reporting to his doctor the numbers that are not "under control" per The Magic Compass Table in Action Step 3. Most importantly, I urged him to consider quitting tobacco use as soon as possible and that I could help him quit when he was ready. He seemed convinced, and he confirmed to me that he would take what I told him seriously.

The Success Story of an 82-Year-Old Man Who Had Diabetes Under Control for 30 Years

In contrast to all of the frightening stories, **clear examples of how favorable lifestyle habits can "positively" impact people's quality of life and prevent all sorts of complications,** are also true to life, as in the numerous people I have counseled, who are now complication-free. One of several such striking examples was a man who was in great shape and who happened to be 82-years-young. He came to the pharmacy and presented prescriptions for an oral diabetes medication. He completely triggered my interest and I started inquiring. After asking him some questions, I had learned from him that he had had diabetes for over 30 years, as he used to be in the past overweight and led a largely sedentary lifestyle. When I asked him about his current blood sugar level, the answer was at his fingertips.

He immediately replied that he checks his sugar levels daily, and that morning, his sugar was 95. (Ideally, it cannot get any better than this). When I asked about his blood pressure, then again, he knew the answer right away and replied that he measures his blood pressure several times a week and records it in a notebook and that it had been consistently at about 125/75. His cholesterol was good, no tingling in his feet whatsoever, signaling that there's no nerve damage or neuropathy, and this was due to his blood sugar being "under control" (below 110).

The only medication he was taking was for diabetes, along with a baby aspirin. I also knew, before he told me and from the great shape he was in, that he must have been leading an active lifestyle. When I inquired about the kinds of activities he did, he replied, "Oh, yes. I walk about an hour a day, and I try to come up with excuses to keep moving around the house." He also replied, "I watch what I eat, and I don't eat too much of anything. Occasionally, I indulge in brownies or ice cream periodically but not all the time.

Ever since I got diabetes some 30 years ago, I took it seriously, lost some weight, watched what I ate; I did just what the doctor told me to do. I started walking and became more active, I take my medications just like I am supposed to, and I check my blood sugar everyday. I have not had a single problem since then." He literally did not leave me room to tell him anything more. He was doing everything right; his lifestyle (and balance) was the key to his healthy life and to his success. I was speechless and could not have said it better myself.

I said "God bless you sir, keep doing what you have been. You look great! I wish all those who have diabetes or don't have diabetes follow in your footsteps." He grinned, thanked me for talking to him, gave me a solid handshake (what a powerful grip he had. I bet if I had a pickle jar at home that I could not open myself, he would have been able to lend me a hand and get it open with his powerful grip) and he walked away. This guy, like many others, is a living example that it can easily be done. This man was happy and seemed to be enjoying life to the fullest. IT IS THAT SIMPLE, AND THAT IS ALL IT TAKES, folks.

In one way or another, the stories I just told you of the people who do not have their diabetes under control are mirrored by almost 90% of diabetics. Some details may differ with each person who has diabetes, but almost all who do not have their diabetes under control can claim that positive lifestyle factors have, undoubtedly, been neglected. Some people may be taking their medications diligently and monitoring their sugar and blood pressure every day, but they're smokers and almost always lead sedentary lifestyles, which explains why their sugar, blood pressure and cholesterol are out of control, "even when they have been taking their medications" regularly. When their life as they know it gets shattered with a massive heart attack or stroke they would seem taken by surprise.

Others may drop off their prescriptions for diabetes, blood pressure and cholesterol at the pharmacy drive-through window, while having a cigarette in their mouth and big bellies bulging out. They have even missed out on the opportunity to make the effort of walking into the pharmacy. As a pharmacist, I despise drive-through windows because it teaches people laziness. I know people with physical disabilities who make the effort to walk into the pharmacy. When I was working at supermarket or discount pharmacy chains, I would have overweight and obese patients come up to the pharmacy counter on a store- provided electric scooter. They drop off their prescriptions for diabetes, cholesterol and high blood pressure and go on driving around effortlessly food shopping.

This is justified for people who have feet and leg problems and if someone has walking limitations and can not walk long distances then making short bouts of 3 or 4 minutes at a time is the answer. But leading a completely sedentary life is not the answer and serves no purpose but fueling the worsening of their chronic conditions. So use the help of the electric scooter in part and when you reach the beginning of the desired aisle then leave the scooter behind and walk to that high fiber cereal box located in the middle of that aisle then try to walk just 30 or 40 seconds more, then you can go back to the scooter for a break. Repeat the same procedure for every item you pick. At the end of an hour or two shopping span you would have benefited from about 10 to 15 minutes of intermittent walking. Not bad for one day. Walking and remaining active as much as our limitations allow us is a must for our own survival

Moreover, the same people who dropped off those prescriptions come back with their basket full of food selections that are totally out-of-balance; snacks that are loaded with refined sugar and bad fat, both of which promote the worsening of their condition and are responsible, in the first place, for disease onset. Their baskets are often loaded with bacon, sausages, white bread, pastas, packages of salty and sweet snacks, butter, margarine, ice cream, marbled meat cuts, jugs of regular soft drinks, hardly any vegetable or fruits, and to top it all off, a carton of cigarettes. The sedentary lifestyles coupled with making unfavorable food choices many people make of course unintentionally and ill informed are major contributing factors to their premature demise and their poor quality of life, due to **debilitating and "preventable" complications.** It is a false sense of security some people have when continuing in the path of faulty lifestyles even if they take their medications. They are not even safe in the haven of their own homes. People can start actually feeling a true sense of security and peace of mind when they start and maintain making *balanced* food and activity choices.

Believe me, I know what overweight and obese people feel and go through because I used to be one myself the first 17 years of my life. It was not easy for me to move around, I was obsessed with food and plagued with making wrong food choices and binging on massive amounts of food. I then lost about 80 pounds of weight in a couple years through strict dieting and deprivation. Then I embarked on a journey shy of three decades to figure out how I could lose weight and maintain that loss, be in control of weight, feel good about myself, be at peace with myself, and prevent disease all without ever dieting again. It took me long years but I set myself free and I found the way. You can too, only it will not take you years to find out what you can do and how you can start developing good habits that help you lose weight and maintain that loss permanently without dieting and deprivation. I have done that search for you.

All you need to know is right here in this guide and in this Action Step 4. I empathize with people going through the same thing I did and my heart goes out to them. I have been doing every thing I can to help people make better lifestyle choices. Keeping the same faulty lifestyle is not the answer. Remaining completely sedentary is not the answer either. Every one can start taking one step at a time forward and this guide in this Action Step 4 will show how. Taking action and regaining control of your health, your weight and your life is the answer and is the way to go forward in this beautiful journey of life. It is never too late. I know every one can do it because as desperate as I was, I did it. There will be solutions for you even with your current

limitations. This Action Step 4 will take you every step of the way. Yes you can do it too, one step at a time. It is that easy.

I can not stress strongly enough that good health **CAN NEVER** be achieved by just taking a pill, but by permanently leading an active and healthy life. It is only by adopting, now, favorable lifestyles choices (as recommended in this section) that you will be able stop the ticking time bomb inside of you. Only you hold the key to that time bomb, and only you can reverse the course of that self-inflicted doomsday. All you need to do is to start taking baby steps, one step at a time, into a better lifestyle. Stop having "a diet mindset," NEVER DIET AGAIN, but start continuously improving your food choices and reducing your portions and when you "mess up," improve your choice next time and keep going.

Finally, if you have lot of stress in your life, find out in the next step, Action Step 5, how you can reduce your stress level, prevent disease complications and regain control of diabetes. Only by taking action now and beginning your journey towards a healthier lifestyle, can you prevent the time bomb from exploding within your own body and within your own home. The only difference between holding onto a grenade after you have taken out the pin and making unfavorable lifestyle choices is the time factor. After you have taken out the pin from that grenade, you will have 6 seconds to dispose of it before it can shatter your world.

By the same token, if you have diabetes, high blood pressure or cardiovascular problems, or if you are overweight and sedentary and/or a smoker or any combination of the above and you don't take any actions now to reverse these trends, then you have already taken the clip out of that lifestyle grenade, and it is only a matter of time before the bomb inside you explodes. My heart saddens greatly when I hear one of my customers tell me that he lost his beloved wife at age 52 who was diabetic and died from a heart attack as a result of out of control diabetes. I feel helpless and guilty at the same time for not having been able to reach out to that man's wife in time in order to help her avoid this tragic end.

It also makes me tremendously sad to know that one of my customer's best friends lost one of her legs at the age of 46 due to diabetes complications. I just cannot look anymore in the sad eyes of a teenager who has lost his precious father who was a diabetic and a smoker and who perished from a massive heart attack at the age of 53. or the sad expressions on the faces of one family of two young daughters, a teenage son and the widow of a 49-year-old man who had high blood pressure from being overweight and who was on dialysis due to complete kidney failure from neglected high blood pressure and who perished from a stroke at age 49. I just cannot see the regret any longer in the eyes of a beautiful 54 year-old-lady, a customer of mine, who suffers from emphysema (a deadly lung disease) and whose companion and best friend is an oxygen bottle and plastic tubing extensions that supply her with artificial oxygen through the nostrils. She has been a smoker for 25 years, and she is obese.

This is not permissible. Millions of similar sad stories are replicated everyday around our country, and they could be entirely preventable. Everyday, thousands of people perish or incur debilitating injuries from the wars they have lost to modifiable lifestyles factors such as smoking; or losses due to not preventing complications that stem from chronic diseases such as diabetes, heart attacks, strokes, amputations, blindness, serious lung diseases and cancer. I know these people exist because I see them every day, I fill their prescriptions and I talk to them; I witness the scars and handicaps from which they have been suffering. If only all of these people had known that their sufferings from all these complications could have been averted, they would have made better choices.

Alarming Obesity Statistics! No Relief in Sight Yet (MUST READ)

This ill-fated trend is continuing, and the end of the catastrophic health crisis that is plaguing our country is not yet in sight. Clear statistical projections and trends are warning that the future decade and beyond could witness, several-fold, the worsening of our state of health; "several-fold worsening" of what we are already suffering from? Oh my!! Recent data from the Centers for Disease Control (CDC) indicated that over a whopping 63 percent of our American population is obese and/or overweight.

The United States is experiencing an explosion in obesity and people suffering from being overweight across the board: all ages, gender, racial and ethnic groups are part of this statistic. Since the last two decades, OBESITY HAS TRIPLED. **The most alarming triple-fold increases are among children and adolescents from the ages of 6-19.** A study released by the U.S. Department of Health and Human Services (HHS), published in *The Journal of the American Medical Association* on March 10, 2004 indicates that premature death due to poor diet (typically Western diet) and physical inactivity (sedentary lifestyle) rose by a staggering 33% in the last 8-10 years. These statistics translate into a sad mortality rate.

The Centers for Disease Control (CDC) reveals startling facts that the yearly preventable premature death toll due to smoking is 472,000 lives, and the yearly preventable premature death toll due to inactivity and obesity is over 433,000 lives. Smoking, obesity, and inactivity cost our nation an estimated 200 billion dollars yearly. **Wow! Over one million people lose their life every year to smoking, obesity and inactivity.** *This is the equivalent of losing, every year, about ten-fold, the US troops lost in all of the 20th century wars combined.*

This means that every second of every day, two people lose their lives prematurely due to modifiable risk factors. Most of all, the priceless mother of all burdens falls on the victim's immediate family members and relatives. **Every day over 130,000 people are grieving a spouse, a mother, a father, a sister, a brother, a son, a daughter, an aunt, an uncle, a grandparent or a friend of a fallen victim who failed to make a choice to stop smoking and/or who failed to make favourable lifestyle choices, quit smoking and lose weight.**

HEALTH RISKS OF OBESITY (MUST READ)

We now know, based on reliable data and clinical trials, that obesity and inactivity cause:

- Premature death
- Type 2 Diabetes (affecting over 20 million people)
- High cholesterol (over 50 million Americans have it)
- Heart Disease
- High Blood Pressure (Over 63 million people have it)
- Stroke
- Blood clots in heart, brain, legs and lungs
- Gall bladder disease
- Varicose veins and swollen legs
- Breathing disturbances while asleep
- Asthma
- Breathing problems (difficulty breathing while performing minimal exertion or walking)
- Fat accumulation inside the tissues of vital organs such as the liver, heart and major arteries, reducing their capacity to function normally

- Cancer (colons, kidneys, endometrial, uterus, breast, prostate and gallbladder)
- Reproductive disorders (women have trouble having children and men have reduced sperm count)
- Menstrual irregularities
- Presence of excess body and facial hair
- Urine leakage caused by weak pelvic muscle
- Complications during surgeries
- Psychological disorders like depression and anxiety
- Stigmatization and discrimination
- Reduced immunity and the capacity to fight off infections
- Catching colds and infections more frequently and taking longer times off work for recovery
- Higher incidences of acid reflux disease and indigestion

If someone is a smoker as well, then the list of fatal risks of smoking is even longer. Similar to obesity, smoking not only has detrimental and damaging effects to the heart, major arteries, blood pressure, blood cholesterol and reproductive organs, but also causes deadly lung diseases and various kinds of cancer including lung cancer. The list goes on and on. It is no secret and no surprise that if someone is overweight, inactive and/or a smoker, and if they continue on this path, their risk of having many of the threats listed above is compounded several-fold.

Unfortunately, the thought that "life-threatening problems happen to others and not me" is rampant, but the crystal clear statistics tell the real story. The risks are so very many that in reality, it is highly likely that you will be inflicted with one or many of these deadly ailments IF you continue on the same path of disregard.

YOU ARE LEFT WITH ONLY ONE CHOICE, AND THE OTHER SIDE OF THE FENCE HAS TO BE GREENER. YOU STILL CAN DO SOMETHING ABOUT YOUR HEALTH, AND IT IS MUCH SIMPLER THAN YOU THINK.

The Good News (MUST READ)

All of these gloomy facts are modifiable!

Lifestyle Choices

Yes this means YOU can change things. **The Centers for Disease Control (CDC) tells us that over 80% of all these illnesses are cause by faulty lifestyle choices. So, this means, if right now you take action and start gradually making better food and activity choices and stop smoking, you can turn these statistics around, all these very serious health threats listed above will stop threatening your safety and your life. You will start enjoying, "right now," the beautiful benefits of good health and best** *quality of life.*

Lisa Wants an Over-the-Counter Diet Pill Recommendation

In my 20 years of experience as a pharmacist, I realized that everybody is looking for good health in a "MAGIC PILL" form that will: offer a cure for all their ailments, provide good health, prevent disease, and promote weight loss. Every week, I receive a number of requests for advice, people asking what the best over-the-counter miracle weight-loss products are. Just yesterday, a beautiful lady, Lisa, who has a weight problem, approached the pharmacy counter with a cute smile on her face and four different over-the-counter weight loss products; she put them on the pharmacy counter and asked, "Which is best of these for weight loss?" I immediately replied that I recommend none of them and that the "Magic Pill" she was looking for is called Lifestyle Choices. She then said that she really "does not have time to exercise" as she baby-sits kids for a living, and she does not go on "Diets" since she had tried many of them and gained the weight right back.

I began to provide Lisa with some tips on various ways she could increase her daily activity and make better food selections. I asked Lisa if she could find 10-15 minutes of free time about 3-4 times per week. She replied affirmatively. I gave her several tips on increasing daily activities by parking away from the store and walking the distance, to always take the longer route while shopping at our store or the local outlets. Then I suggested she would schedule every other day, one half hour session or two fifteen minute bouts of brisk walking (brisk meaning a speed faster than her normal walking pace); or she could choose stationary cycling or any other favourite activity. I also suggested she wear padded walking shoes for comfort and injury prevention.

For food, I suggested she increase her fiber intake by selecting foods such as: whole grain, oatmeal, beans, vegetables, fruits and told her to consume 3 main meals and 2 fruit snacks per day. We also talked about reducing portion sizes and switching regular soft drinks to water and diet soft drinks. She seemed satisfied and promised to take action. As she was leaving the pharmacy counter, her extremely obese teenage daughter met up with her. I felt really sad that such a young girl who could not have been more than 17 and who weighed no less than 290 pounds, would most likely be facing, soon, a number of health challenges unless she made radical changes to her lifestyle choices right away.

The Media Shoving Ridiculously "Thin" Models in Our Faces As Symbols of "Good Health"

People have misconceptions about various health-related issues as they get bombarded with conflicting and inaccurate information from the media. A myriad of advertisements promote "quick weight loss" with fad diets or fad diet pills; these ads promote thinness by showing tip-top models with flawless bodies. The purpose of permanent weight loss and weight management is not to become thin, but rather to have a better quality of life, to prevent disease and disease complications, and to have a better self-image. Lifelong good health can NEVER be a quick fix or a part time hobby that is achievable by popping pills or following a diet that restricts certain food categories or that starts on a Monday and ends on a Friday, three or more months later.

Lifelong good health is a full-time commitment, and it can be non-restrictive, flexible, and fun. By the same token, permanent weight loss and weight management is an everyday commitment where you make balanced food and activity choices and make a consistent effort to improve these choices and to never feel that you have "failed." When you "mess up," you did not fail; you just decided to controllably indulge, and you should, occasionally when you feel like it. You fail when you aim for perfection and you are too rigid and hard on yourself. Just make a better choice next time.

The damage that these quick-fix diets and fad diet pills have created is that they are restrictive and can be difficult to follow long-term, so people who use them, lose and regain the weight in a yoyo manner. The same applies to diet pills where the manufacturer promises weight loss even when users "eat all the food they want to and don't have to exercise." This relieves the user's responsibility of adopting favourable lifestyle choices. The same applies to people who request and get prescriptions for diet and fluid pills from their doctor. At the pharmacy checkout, they will purchase their diet pills but they are also buying a big bag of mozzarella cheese sticks, a large bag of marshmallows, soft candy, chocolate bars, regular sodas; and they snack on them all day! These processed packaged snacks consist of pure sugar, salt, and Trans Fats (artery-clogging fat) these are the very same ingredients that cause weight gain and trigger hunger, which make you want to eat more.

Chris, an Overweight Pharmacy Technician, Wonders Why He Cannot Lose Weight

During pharmacy practice, I watched, diligently, the patterns of customers and co-workers alike. In any store at which I worked, I have "never" seen "any" of the technicians or cashiers with whom I worked, snack on fruits or vegetables. Their meals consisted of fatty fried foods with loads of bread, fried rice or pasta or other nutrient-deficient foods such as packaged saltines, chips, candy and cookies. I hardly saw any of my co-workers sips on water, but regularly sipped on their favourite sugar-laden soft drinks or juices. It seemed I was the only one bringing plenty of fruits and veggies, and I pushed everyone around me to consume more of these nutrient-dense foods.

The most interesting part of these scenarios is that those same people, who were downing these foods, were constantly wondering "why" they kept gaining weight or why they weren't able to lose any. One recent example of this type of scenario includes a highly skilled technician in South Texas. It had been fun working that store since we joked around all the time, though we worked hard, at the while. He was sharp, very efficient and fast. His name is Chris. Chris was a 26 year-old man who'd been married for five years and had a very beautiful 2-year-old-daughter and a lovely wife.

Chris however, was overweight. From watching his lifestyle patterns, I could tell why. A typical daily breakfast, which he got from the local donut shop, consisted of a couple of large sausage pastries and a large glazed donut. For lunch, he might have two large fast-food burgers laden with mayo and cheese and a super-sized order of fries, and a large regular soda. He had an inconsistent eating pattern, in the sense that he skipped meals, thinking he was doing well; and then he'd make up for that missed meal with a large candy bar. In terms of activity, he led, largely, a sedentary lifestyle. If Chris does not make a decision to start taking small steps towards a more favorable lifestyle, he will undoubtedly develop one or more of the deadly chronic conditions listed in the "Risks of Overweight & Obesity" section above. He will become a statistic just like the tens of millions of Americans battling the ailments of obesity and diabetes; this means his cute little daughter will have to grow up witnessing "Daddy" battle a deadly chronic disease (or worse) unless he takes action NOW and starts taking baby steps in the right direction.

Identifying Barriers and Finding Solutions
With Favorable Lifestyle Choices

Ask yourself, "What makes me not want to take action now and start changing my life for the better?" Here are some common barriers that many people claim:

- **"I have no time."** Solution: If this is your answer because you work long hours and you have to juggle responsibilities between home, work and family then you and millions like you have legitimate time issues, you have my full respect and understanding because believe me I can relate with my 80 hour work weeks. Not making changes to the better in your lifestyle is no excuse either and no you do not have to diet and you do not have to go out of your way to "exercise." Remember your good health is so precious and that is what is enabling you juggle all these responsibilities.

- Without your good health you will not be able to juggle anything. So here is the solution. Regarding food intake, all you need is to preplan and make more favorable food selections, starting from your weekly supermarket trips and take these high fiber snacks with you to work and learn how to make healthier food choices when you eat out without affecting the quality or taste of food. This will be discussed in detail in the next upcoming food section and you will have lots of tips at your disposal and you will generate your own ideas as well. Regarding activity, you do not need to be going to the gym for two hours a session in order to benefit; but rather, the gym is everywhere you are. Increase the amount of walking you do at work, home and while shopping. For more tips on this, check out "Tips on How to Increase Daily Activity" in the activity section.

- **"I have no willpower necessary to lose weight."** Solution: You don't need any. You are not starting a diet and you are not expected to muster all your effort to remain without a certain food for any period of time, and you are not required to run in the next marathon. All that is required from you is to make better food and activity choices, and when you "mess up," make a better choice the next time, and you will notice that the more you exercise your ability to make good choices, that your choices will regularly keep improving.

- **"I have failed before, and I am tired of trying to lose weight."** Solution: Name one person in our Universe (The Earth and surrounding planets) who has not failed in one way or another. Success comes after failure and he bigger the failure, the bigger the success. The glass is always half full. Though losing weight and keeping it off is no simple matter, those who have succeeded kept trying until they won. Those who have control over their weight have dropped the "diet" concept. See the section "The Habits of

People Who Lost Weight and Kept It Off" which you will find later in this section.

- **"I have no money. I am on a fixed budget."** Solution: You do not need any additional money. There is no need for gym membership, no need to invest in equipment, no need to blow your budget on expensive "Quick Weight Loss" products or "diet club" memberships. All you need to do is to make better food selections at the supermarket, at home, while eating out and at work, as will be discussed in the food section. For more activity tips check out the activity section further down.

- **"I'm not athletic. I don't like to exercise."** Solution: No one is asking you to be athletic or to love exercising. If you notice, I have not used the word exercise in this guide for fear of discouraging those who "don't like to exercise." There are misconceptions about how much activity is needed for good health and weight loss. Actually, not much is needed. Just increase your total activity and walking intermittently to about 30 or 45 minutes daily as will be discussed in the activity section. You can accomplish anything you want.

In this upcoming section, I will mention 3 habits; if you adopt them and apply them, they will transform your health and life.

Learn How to Build New Good Habits

The 3 Habits that Will Transform Your Health and Life (MUST READ)

- Persistence
- Balance
- Variety

Persistence

Whatever you do in life, if you do not take any action or series of actions regarding any specific goal or task, then you cannot achieve your objective. There are situations that come up during anyone's life that sometimes require immediate action or a sustained series of actions for a prolonged period of time. For example, let's say you are at home or at work and a fire breaks out in the room you are in, and the fire is blocking the exit door. You know that in that room, there are two windows that could lead you to safety. So what actions do you take? Of course, you want to rescue yourself. Within seconds, the smoke fills the room and visibility is nil. So you find your way to the first window; it's completely shut, and you cannot open it. So what do you do?

At this stage, the smoke has filled the room, and the fire is very near. Are you moving slowly like you are taking a walk in the park? or are you just standing there, taking no action? Neither. You move frantically and fast, scanning and feeling your way to all possible exits. If one is blocked, then you rush to the other and keep **persistently trying** until you find the next window; you break it and free yourself from DANGER. Was inaction, at any time, an option in that inferno? Your life was in danger. You took action by persistently trying other options until you succeeded and freed yourself from that danger. Inaction was "never" an option. Yet, in real life, tens of millions of people in the U.S. choose inaction and are virtually "staying in that room and doing nothing." I take that back, they are actually staying in that room, but unintentionally they are feeding the fire and making it worse. **The toll? ONE MILLION LIVES EVERY YEAR ARE CLAIMED BY OBESITY, INACTIVITY AND SMOKING. How so, you ask?**

When people who have diabetes, high cholesterol, heart disease or high blood pressure come to the pharmacy, drop off their prescriptions for an antibiotic or their prescriptions for diabetes, cholesterol and/or heart medications, then turn around and order a triple-decker cheeseburger slathered with mayo and grease, along with a super-sized soda, then finish their meal off with a cigarette and go home and sit in front of the tube for six long hours watching TV, would these people be feeding the fire in that room or not?

Now, here is another example of persistence. Anyone can think back to any new job or position you really wanted and got. First, you knew you had to "act" (persistent action) by going to that interview and trying to impress your interviewer with your credentials. You get accepted to that position, and then what do you do? You "act" again (persistent action) by learning the work place requirements, and you act yet again by learning and training yourself on the various tasks assigned to you. For the first three or four weeks or more, you "act" (persistent action) by learning your new tasks.

At first, if you think back, were you very comfortable initially with your new assignments? Did you know and execute everything required from you flawlessly? or rather, did it take you some time (a series of persistent and repetitive actions of errors and corrections over a period of several weeks) until you were able to master all the tasks required from you? Having good health as we age is paramount. **If you are a smoker and do nothing (no persistent actions), you will most likely end up like Peter Jennings of ABC and George Harrison of The Beatles.**

But, on the other hand, if you execute a series of persistent actions in favor of your health, such as: learning to build a habit of making better food choices; and building a habit of walking more each day by making more frequent trips; and learning to take the longer way during your several daily errands and chores, that would be like the persistent actions you took to learn the new tasks assigned to you in that job. Would your small but "persistent" actions to quit smoking or lose weight by taking more steps each day and by learning to make better food choices in order to improve diabetes, blood pressure and cholesterol control benefit your health?

From now on, failure is your friend; because when you are trying, you might fail at times, but you will learn from those failures. With persistent repetition, you get yourself a favorable habit for a lifetime. And that deserves congratulations. Those who tried and failed in their attempt to quit smoking or to lose weight, and who "kept on" trying after that initial failure, have actually prevailed. So, when you are faced with a problem, think of the smoke in that room. Keep trying until you find another solution. Every problem and obstacle has several solutions. Smoking and obesity are formidable foes and killers (major threats like the fire and smoke in that room). When you are faced with a challenge, come up with several solutions and act on them, and remain persistent with your quest to achieve better health for life and you will prevail. You "can" choose favorable actions for your health; you are worth it. Remember, if you have good health, the possibilities are endless.

Balance

Well, the word balance is the opposite of perfection. Moreover, balance in food intake is the opposite of food deprivation and gigantic portion sizes. *Nobody* is perfect, or will there ever be anybody who is perfect. The only perfect being is God. And to equate yourself with God and perfection will surely bring you disappointment, because, in essence we are human. **Balance is similar to being FLEXIBLE. Also, balance is the opposite of extreme action: overdoing, inflexible or rigid actions and expectations.** This means that if you are aiming for perfection, exaggerated actions and "all-or-none" behavior, you can only last for a short period of time, and then you are doomed for failure. Aim at making more balanced choices only 80% of the time. Only then are you able to last indefinitely, since you are not being deprived of anything and your mind will sense that. **If you make small and "persistent" balanced actions that promote good health, then you will have built yourself favorable habits for a lifetime.**

The "all-or-none" perfectionist and exaggerated behavior will have the same result that occurs with your New Year's resolutions; in about three weeks into the new year, you usually drop everything you started and go back to square one. Does a diet seem like a perfectionist's approach or a balanced action that anyone can maintain for life? Is that diet approach a likely "permanent" solution? Maybe not. A more balanced approach would be to first drop the perfectionist "dieting" mindset because it leads to failure. Then start aiming at eating three main meals from all the food groups, but in smaller portions, as recommended in the food section further down.

Do not super-size anything (this will be an exaggerated and a non balanced action when you choose extra large portion sizes) Include two fruit or veggie snacks in between meals, and cut back on all sweetened or salty packaged snacks as they contain no nutritional value but contribute greatly to weight gain. Switch from regular soda to diet soft drinks or water. In terms of activity, make an effort to increase your amount of walking gradually when you are at work, at the store, at home or shopping. Practice taking the longer way, and three times a week, schedule walking or any favorite outdoor or indoor activity such as treadmill, cycling, or swimming for 30 minutes at a pace faster than your normal pace.

So how does balance and persistence factor in here? Say you have succeeded most of the week at eating small-portion sizes, then the weekend came and you were at a party and you indulged in chips and cheeses? Then cake and chocolate came along and you ate a hefty portion of the cake and could not resist that chocolate! You wake up the next day, you feel guilty because you think you "messed up" or "failed" your diet, and you decide to give it all up. Not yet pal, hold your horses.

Well first of all, remember that you were not dieting, then remember that you made good food choices most of the week, almost 80% of that week, and you have been more active than before; so this is the 20% part where you can indulge in a controllable manner. So give yourself a pat on the back and don't feel guilty not one bit. The persistence is mandatory to overcoming that obstacle continue making and improving your lifestyle choices. **Remember, making better food choices is not like switching an "on and off" button, but it is a process that you must improve on regularly and persistently.**

Variety

If you eat the same food day in and day out, and if you choose the same walking route and the same activity every day for a while, then you fall into a rut; soon, you start thinking of dropping the whole thing and going back to your "I'm sitting on the couch, watching the game, so hand me the beer and chips, and don't me get up" set of habits.

Better yet, consuming a variety among all foods ensures that you are getting all the nutrients your body needs. There is no one food, meat, fruit or vegetable that contains all the nutrients you need. But when you include a ***balanced variety from all favorable food choices*** (as discussed in the food section) in ***balanced portion sizes***, a variety of cooking methods (not only frying) and a variety of cuisines, whether you eat in or out, then you will be making sure that you are consuming a wide variety of nutrients that contribute to your good health. Also these balanced food choices will help you end the hunger cycle, lose weight and keep it off, keep your blood sugar levels "under control," reduce your cholesterol and prevent heart disease (examples of foods that lower cholesterol and help prevent heart disease are: the good oils such as olive oil, the Omega 3' oils found in almonds, walnuts and fish (such as salmon, tuna, sardines, and other types of fish). (See an extensive list in the food section).

As to activity, variety is essential and crucial for growth and improvement. If you do the same activity every time, for prolonged periods, then your muscles, heart, lungs, and blood circulation are not challenged for further gain. But by adopting a "variety" approach, you stimulate your body to respond and progress, and you **boost your capacity to go beyond that weight loss plateau.**

Now you realize that in order for anyone to reap lifelong good health and lose and be in control of their weight permanently, they need to be **persistent** in improving their **balanced** actions in terms of food and activity choices. This means avoiding a "perfectionist," "deprivation" and "overdoing-it" approach. Top off the "persistent," "balanced" and "flexible" approach with **variety** in your food and activity selection (and really, in any aspect of your life); **it is then and only then that you can permanently**

regain control over your weight, health and any other aspect of your life. NEVER DIET AGAIN.

Armed with these three powerful and simple concepts, you can build favorable habits of your choosing that last a lifetime. Some exceptions to the balanced approach is smoking or using tobacco products or using illegal drugs. Remember smoking is a formidable danger. You need to get away from it, as far as possible, and immediately. No halfway solutions there.

Unlock the Secrets of How to Develop New and Favorable Habits And Regain Unlimited Control Over Your Life and Health

WHAT IS A HABIT?

Can we undo bad habits such as smoking or making unfavorable food choices, and build new favorable lifestyle habits?

The word "habit" has come up a lot, but what is actually a habit and what is it's significance on our health? Any *small* action that is *not exaggerated*, good or bad, that you repeat many times daily and weekly for about three weeks becomes a habit. An example of a good action that could become a favorable habit is the one I gave in the "Persistence" section about starting a new job. If you recall, in that example, when you first started that job, everything seemed awkward and out of place. The computer software system that you needed to learn was not easy at first. But you learned to apply it (persistent action) a bit at a time (small steps) each day, and after about three to four weeks (repeated small actions) you became very comfortable with that software as if it were second nature (habit). When you occasionally messed up, you were coached, you corrected that mistake and kept going (You made an error, learned from it, you moved on and did not quit).

If you apply this same concept to building new and favorable lifestyle habits, such as increasing activity and reducing portion sizes of foods consumed, you can apply the exact same pattern. Just like that job you did not feel comfortable with at first, and you did not learn all the tasks assigned to you in one day; but you made small repeated actions, (persistence + balanced actions), and followed through with correction of errors and learning new tasks, until everything became easy after three or so weeks. Only after going through this initial period, were you able to perform most of those tasks without looking at manuals or notes and without being coached by anyone. **This has become your new habit**. So you took about three or four weeks to build a solid base and foundation for your long-term career goal. The same applies with regard to favorable lifestyle choices.

John Doe's Current Habits: A Typical "Eat, Sit and Smoke Like There Is No Tomorrow" Kind of Day

John you have been diabetic for quite some time; you are a smoker, thrive on a "Western Diet" and lead a typical sedentary lifestyle. Let us consider a day that describes your current lifestyle, according to what you told me at the pharmacy-counseling window.

You get up in the morning, skip breakfast and drive to work. You park in the very first parking spot, take the elevator to your office on the second floor, sit for several hours behind your desk and perform your work duties until lunch time. You take the elevator down to your car (missed an opportunity to walk a small bout and expand energy), drive to the local fast food restaurant, order your typical "Western Diet" meal: a double-decker bacon cheeseburger with mayo and butter on the bread, fries, and a 16 ounce regular soda.

The clerk offers to super size (twice the quantity) everything for "ONLY" 39 cents more (the cheapest way to send you to the hospital emergency room, suffering from a heart attack or a stroke sooner rather than later, and you incur major expenses, and you blow your quality of life; that is if you are still alive, all for only 39 cents. What a bargain!!).

You gulp down that entire feast; as you leave, you light up a cigarette, you get in your car and you head back to work. You attempt to park in your same first spot (avoiding more opportunity to walk and expand energy) next to the entrance (and not a foot away). Unfortunately, your spot has been taken. You are furious at this point, and right before you call the wrecker service to have this car that took your assigned spot, the closest spot to your destination, towed away, the owner arrives and is about to pull out.

You finally breathe a sigh of relief and you put your blinker on and wait, wait some more, for a whole 5 minutes to reclaim your spot, knowing that 3 spots up (a little farther away from the entrance which requires more walking, of course) there were plenty of parking spaces. Finally, you get back to your office and you sit for several more hours

(Conserving more energy and gaining more weight) the rest of the evening at your desk, working again. Mid-afternoon hunger strikes, so you are at the mercy of vending machines you eat a couple of packages of peanut butter crackers or Twinkies full of artery-clogging Trans Fatty acids and sugar.

The workday comes to an end, you get in your car and go to pick up the kids from school by driving as close to the pick-up area as possible, then you drive to the pharmacy to pick up your diabetes medications, pull to the drive through window with a cigarette dangling from your mouth. The pharmacist counsels you on the prescriptions you are filling and suggests strongly that you quit smoking, and when he suggests you become more active, since activity is so vital to controlling your condition, your reply, of course, is "I don't have time."

You head home, and for dinner you eat pizza with the works, of course "meat lovers pizza" stacked with pepperoni, sausage, the whole works. Of course, you "wash down" that pizza with a "couple beers" (amassing an enormous amount of dense and fatty foods that contribute to weight gain and heart disease.

Now it is activity time, you literally walk the whole distance from the dining room to the living room, then you (guessed right) sit on your favorite couch, puff on a couple of cigarettes and watch TV for the rest of the night. And Oh! Let's not forget a small piece of dessert before the night is over ("just" a wedge of cheesecake topped with whipped cream and maybe a large scoop or two of double fudge chocolate ice cream).

In summary of your lifestyle, you sit, sit, sit, eat enormous amounts of fatty, salty and sugar-loaded foods, smoke, sit, eat some more, smoke, sit, and sit some more, eat, smoke, sit and then sleep. Did I understand your inquiry correctly, at the pharmacy drive-through window, that you are wondering why your doctor cannot get your sugar, cholesterol and blood pressure levels under control? You also said that you don't have time to walk a bit more every day!!

These have been John's current habits. He arrived at this lifestyle due to repeated faulty actions over the years. These accumulated faulty actions have become his new behavior and now fully define his lifestyle, which in his unknowing, is putting him in harm's way. His life will be in serious and grave danger "soon" unless he chooses to have a complete lifestyle makeover.

Can any of you readers relate to this story in one way or another? I know you can, because in my pharmacy practice, I have witnessed you doing some of these things, in one way or another. I have watched what's in your plates when you order food at the food courts of that pharmacy where you drop off your prescriptions for diabetes, cholesterol, blood pressure, and heart disease or for all of them. I have also seen what is in your food-shopping cart. This, of course, has been the description of a typical day, more or less, one that millions of Americans go through day after dangerous day, but of course with individual variations.

Maybe some do not have kids or a desk job. Maybe some are not smokers. But largely and for the most part, people are thriving on the "Western Lifestyle" and the kind of life it espouses: watching too much TV, leading sedentary lifestyles, top that off with a "Western Diet" and such eating patterns that consist of **mega portions** of burgers, fries, regular soda, pizzas, hot dogs, ice cream, cheese cakes, cookies, packaged snacks, and other "junk food." Just like John. For whatever reason, you seem to be locked in a negative unfavorable lifestyle loop that you think you cannot get out of. I tell you that **YOU CAN** while still enjoying the foods you like and that you grew up with but with small modification of portion sizes and food choices.

If you think about it, you did not develop these unfavorable habits in a day or two. You have made unfavorable selections (actions), one at a time (small increments) over a period of time (repetition) until the sum of all these unfavorable food selections and inactivity have become a part of your daily pattern (habits). Now, likewise, it is time to reverse this trend for your betterment in small increments and one step at a time into a positive and favorable lifestyle.

Now what was the definition of a habit? Any action, good or bad, that you repeat many times daily and weekly becomes a habit after about three weeks. Any action, good or bad, that is.

This means we are not born with habits but, rather, we have the direct input in choosing those that we want to be part of our lifestyle. However, people will never become perfect, and we shouldn't set ourselves up for failure by thinking that we can become "perfect." So if you sometimes make "bad" choices, you are not the only one. We all do. But what you can and should also choose to include are some good choices in your lifestyle most of the time, as well. In the same manner that people can include bad habits in their lifestyle, like overeating, inactivity and smoking, they can also learn to include good ones as well, such as making more balanced food and activity choices.

Believe it or not, when you include good habits in your lifestyle, you can undo bad ones such as smoking and overeating. You are in control now. You can include any favorable habit in your lifestyle, but just remember how you can do that:

MUST READ:
The Key to Building Favorable Habits for a Lifetime:

1. Repeat desired action daily and weekly (hopefully it is a favorable action for your health that you are choosing).
2. Improve choices, and when you "mess up," don't quit; don't be a perfectionist, but do better next time and just keep going.
3. Allow 3-4 weeks of repeating that action in order for it to become a habit.

RESULT: You have built yourself a new lifestyle pattern, or in other words, a new "habit."

After 3 or 4 weeks, that new habit becomes a part of your lifestyle. The more you do it, the more it feels like it's been there forever. Just like that new job example in the "persistence" section above, after 3-4 weeks, everything becomes easier and falls into place. You don't have to look for the stapler because you know where it is. It is in the 3rd drawer, so you reach for it and get it. When you get a glitch on your computer, you don't ask for help or look in your notes. You now know how to resolve it yourself, without help. From that point on, everything becomes first nature. Then you go to work, day after day, and you can find everything and perform every task effortlessly, as if you have been there forever.

The same applies to new habits you are trying to introduce to your lifestyle such as making balanced food choices and trying to do more walking every day. The first 3-4 weeks, you try to make those choices, sometimes you succeed in remembering that new action and sometimes you forget. No big deal. So you improve your choices every time (just like the first few weeks on that new job); but you keep repeating your actions. Soon, you start making better choices, most of the time, and after 3-4 weeks, you start remembering to make that extra walking loop at the supermarket, and you select whole grain bread without forgetting, and when you are asked to super-size your burger order, you decline the offer, you ask for a diet soft drink instead of the regular because now you like the taste better than the regular one, and you substitute your "mayo" with mustard, and you request dry bread, not drenched with butter.

Most importantly, you start making these choices without hesitation and without forgetting, because now (after 3-4 weeks of "training"), everything is coming together; and you can go on permanently doing this because you are not dieting anymore, and you are not deprived of any food groups. Whenever you feel like eating ice cream or fries, you are the master of your choices; you can have those fries and the ice cream, but in smaller quantities than before, and less frequently per week, because now, most of the time, you have been selecting high-fiber foods as listed in detail in the food section next, and you have balanced out the consumption of other food groups as well.

Moreover, you have increased your level of activity several-fold, and everywhere you go, you park further away, and you make the extra effort of walking (during every errand and every chore you do, and you have tremendously increased the number of chores you are doing, daily).

It all starts coming together; you start losing weight right away, and you keep it off; you start feeling better about yourself. Most importantly, as the ultimate result of all your positive choices that you have been making most of time, you bring your diabetes, cholesterol and blood pressure under control and you move away from you the constant threat of deadly complications that was aimed at the heart of you. These have become your new behaviors and your new habits, which you are able to maintain for a lifetime because they are balanced, and you do not experience a sense of deprivation. **It is that simple. Anyone can do it, you need NOT any will power and you do not have to become an athlete to have good health.**

Try This at Home—Simple Proof that Anyone Can Learn a Good New Habit and Unlearn a Bad One at the Same Time

Let's put this to the test right now. Lay down this guide and cross your arms. It is natural and simple right? Now cross them the opposite way. Less straightforward and uncomfortable, isn't it? If you practice crossing your arms the opposite way several times daily, in about three weeks this task becomes a piece of cake. In other words, when you cross your arms from that point on, in the opposite way, it becomes natural and second nature to you; that's because you practiced daily and weekly, crossing your arms in that opposite way, until it became simpler and it became a **habit**.

Here is another simple example. Go to the drawer in your kitchen where your utensils are. Take the forks out and put them in your pantry, and leave them there for a couple of days. When it is time for your next meal, notice where you are going to go first to find the forks. Of course, the former spot and when you get there, you will remember that you put them in the pantry. In fact, you will automatically go to the former spot several times before you start heading first to the pantry. When you **learn the new habit** (which is the new location in the pantry) **you unlearn** the previous location. But with repeated actions and corrections of the mix-ups, you will go to the right location, immediately, several trials later. Simply put, you have just developed a new habit by repeating your actions and correcting and learning from your mistakes.

John Doe's Attempt to Have a Lifestyle Makeover

The same habit-forming rule needs to apply when it comes to making favorable lifestyle choices in terms of food and activity selections. So let's rewind above to John Doe's story of a typical day and see how we can help him make better choices which will help him lose weight and regain permanent control of his diabetes and of his life, "without" dieting.

John, before you can start making favorable lifestyle choices, some pre-planning would have to take place. Always wear comfortable broken in rubber-padded shoes for the extra walking. Do some pre-planning by going to the supermarket for food shopping. You need to shop for vegetables, fruits, whole grain breads, lean meats, fish and seafood canned or fresh beans, oat bran or oatmeal and high fiber cereal AND DEVELOP A HABIT OF READING LABELS. For a balanced snack tip see "Become a Nutrition Label" before the "Meal Structure Blueprint" few sections below. Bring them home, wash the fruit and vegetables and prepare them so you can take them as a snack for the next day.

Now, I assume that preplanning has already taken place and snack arsenals from what you brought home such as fruits, vegetables, vegetable dips, mixed nuts and high fiber cereal are ready to go.

You get up in the morning, you make extra walking trips inside the house between your bedroom, bathroom and the kitchen, you walk up and down the steps a couple of times to get things, making one walking trip per chore, for a total of 3-4 minutes. Then you head to the kitchen, you won't skip breakfast this time; you will have a bowl of **great tasting** high-fiber cereal, such as Kashi or FiberOne brands, along with low fat milk or soymilk. If you are Lactose intolerant then choose the Lactose free milk or soymilk.

You take along the snacks and you drive to work where you park your car in the very furthest spot; this gives you a chance to walk a little more. Instead of taking the elevator this time, you take the stairs to the first floor, then the elevator to the second floor (a week later you can walk up the stairs to the second floor; remember, John, not to overdo, but to take a balanced and gradual approach to increase the amount of activity that you do daily. If your work is in the 56th story please don't be walking up or down 56 floors. Instead you can take the elevator to the 53rd floor and walk the steps up 3 more stories to your office. You can do the same on the way down and in smaller buildings).

Once in the office, you do not delegate any task requiring movement or activity to anyone, but you make the effort yourself. Also, make one trip for each task; do not make one trip for every three or four tasks. For example if you need to make copies for some documents, want to get some water (**sipping on 6 to 8 glasses of water daily is essential**), and the last task being a trip to the restroom. Instead of doing all three tasks in one trip, make a trip for each of them and then return back to your desk each time. First, go to the restroom, then come back to your desk via the longer route; afterwards, take the documents to your assistant to copy or copy it yourself. Then return to your desk. A little later, go get some water, then return back to your desk, of course taking the longer way.

You can be creative within your own environment and come up with ideas to make more frequent errands. Having said that, you know what limitations you have in your own work place, so use commonsense. If you are short on time and are running behind then by all means do 20 tasks in the same trip. Maybe increasing activity at a specific period of time during work is not appropriate then do whatever works. Despite all the work limitations, everyone can creatively and without affecting their work flow, increase their daily walking in the work environment by at least 30 to 50%. After all, healthy employees use less sick days and they are much more productive on the job than their less healthy counterparts.

It is midmorning now, and you are feeling a bit hungry. You are no more at the mercy of vending machines because your pre-planning (by going to the supermarket) has paid off and has come to your rescue. To your colleagues' surprise, you pull out the banana that you brought with you from home, along with a teaspoon of peanut butter or a pinch of nuts or a bite of your favorite Belgian dark chocolate (remember, you are practicing reducing portion sizes along with favorable food and snack selection).

FOR THE CURIOUS ONLY

When you combine fruit with proteins, good sources of fat or fiber (like John is doing when combining a banana with nuts or dark chocolate), the sugar in the fruit will be metabolized at a slower pace and causes only a moderate rise of blood sugar and consequently lesser insulin is produced. *In simple terms, you don't get hungry as fast.*

After the brief snack, you proceed with your workload at the office and continue your quest to increase your activity. Another tip on increasing your activity at work, John, is adopting "the 4 foot rule" which is placing frequently used items, such as pens stapler, trash can etc. at a 3 or 4 foot radius away from you. As a consequence you get to make more frequent trips in the process. (See the Activity section of Action Step 4 for more details).

Now it is lunchtime, so you take the stairs down instead of the elevators. If the restaurant is within walking distance, then you dump the car and you walk. If it is raining, then you take the umbrella along and you walk. If it is far, then you take the car along and you park in the last spot, as usual, at that fast food restaurant lot. Now, instead of ordering your typical "Western Diet" meal, you skip that double-decker bacon-burger and you make a wiser choice this time. You order the regular hamburger combo meal or grilled chicken combo meal. Now tell the cashier to substitute mayo with mustard and/or catsup, and to not use butter on the bread. Better yet, ask if whole grain bread is available and request it. All else in that burger, including lettuce and tomato remain unchanged.

Your Tastes Buds Can Adapt to New Tastes

If you are craving cheese, then listen to your craving so you don't feel as if you've been cheated you can add cheese (but then alternate choices and try to order the burger without cheese next time, to create a balanced approach). For your drink, request a diet soda, water or iced tea sweetened with Splenda or other sugar substitutes. You might now be thinking,

"I don't like the taste of diet soda." I will tell you again, that taste is adaptable. Try diet soda for about a week, and then taste the regular soda again. I will bet you that you will dislike the taste of regular soft drinks. Your taste buds will adapt to the new taste. Likewise, once you start eating foods with lower content of sugar and grease then your taste buds will adapt too. So after consuming these less dense foods and you taste again those greasy foods then you will notice the difference and wonder how were you able to eat them all the time. All sweeteners are safe for human consumption but see the Warning statement on page 167 titled "Sweeteners" if you are pregnant and about a substance called Phenylalanine found in many sweeteners containing Aspartame.

If you have only been drinking one 12-oz regular soda a day, then by making the switch to the diet soda (many people drink a whole lot more), you will lose about 11 pounds per year (by taking this action alone). Recent statistics show that overweight people may consume, on average, 16-32 ounces of regular soda a day. You do the math.

Now the cashier is asking you whether you want to super-size your order for ONLY 39 CENTS more. Of course, you will decline her offer to super-size a heart attack for only 39 cents. But you are not done ordering yet. Don't forget to order a side garden salad with your favorite dressing. You could order a light dressing if the taste is doable. Otherwise, use half to one packet of your regular favorite dressing with your salad and skip the croutons and bacon bits since there is enough bread and fat in your burger and fries. Now your order is complete.

Of course you wonder, what about the fries, is it taboo or not? Remember you are not on a "diet" and you will NOT eliminate any food but you can eat anything in a balanced manner. So eat the fries, if you want to, and don't have an ounce of guilt since you have made favorable modifications to your order and have not super-sized your order and you have skipped the butter, Mayo, croutons and bacon bits. Since you will be trying to practice a balanced lifestyle approach, you might try to limit eating fries to once or twice a week without super-sizing it.

So, you get your order, and since you are eating fries, it is a good idea to shave off some of the burger bread, around the circumference of the top and lower part of the burger buns. Now, you have successfully modified a typical "Western Diet" meal and customized it to fit your current and more favorable lifestyle and approach to healthy eating.

As a variation, if you feel like having cheese on your burger and eating all the bread on the burger, then let go of the fries (or onion rings). To vary your meal options, next time, when having lunch, choose another non-fast-food restaurant. **This modification for that meal has helped you slash about 40 to 50% of unnecessary food overage which could help you lose about 8 to 10 pounds per year with substitutions of 1 to 2 similar meals per week over the course of a whole year.**

Of course, if you eat out more frequently and you make more similar substitutions several times a week, then you have the potential to lose a lot more weight per year, and that loss is permanent, *if you keep the same lifestyle and positive food choices.*

So you complete the meal and walk out to your car, only this time, you don't light up a cigarette because you have quit smoking by using my "Stop Smoking Now" guide or other smoking cessation literature and programs offered by reputable health associations such the American Cancer Society and the American Heart Association. So, you drive back to your office, and again you park in the last spot in that lot, you walk through the lot and you skip the elevator and you take the steps to your office, continuing all the while to come up with ideas to walk some more and run more errands the rest of the day till 6:00 p.m. comes, your quitting time.

At about 4:30 p.m., it is time for your mid-afternoon snack. So you get the mixed nuts that you brought with you from home and you eat a pinch full followed by your favorite fruit or maybe some broccoli, celery or cucumber along with the vegetable dip you brought with you from home. **This mid-day snack is essential and must not be skipped because it gives you a load of nutrients and energy that allows you to get home and not be hungry. Because you are not hungry, you do not raid the refrigerator, and you end up doing 20 to 30 minutes on your stationary bicycle before dinner without "starving to death."**

You get off work and take the stairs down to your car, parked further down that lot. Then you head to school, pick up your kids. Only now you park your car at the beginning of the block and you walk to meet your kids at the school pick-up site; or if they are within sight, you let them walk to you so they can do their share of taking extra steps too. Now you drive to the pharmacy to pick up your diabetes medications. Forget the drive-through. Park your car in a distant part of the parking lot and take your kids along and take advantage of this brief walking and bonding moment, and pick up your medications from the pharmacy counter. You are no longer buying cigarettes because you quit since you realized how detrimental tobacco is to your health and to managing your diabetes.

Now, you drive home and there you quickly change from work clothes to walking gear clothes and shoes. You hop on your stationary bicycle and you cycle for about 20 to 30 minutes while catching the latest game scores or the latest news on TV. You are now a healthy role model for your kids who are watching you cycle instead of watching you smoke or sit.

Then you shower and it's time for a delicious meal. Instead of pizza, you will have blackened fish with lemon served with vegetables sautéed in olive oil, along with kidney beans prepared with lemon and olive oil dressing and garnished with sautéed almonds (double doses of Omega 3).

Of course, don't forget drinking 6 to 8 glasses of water during the day, with meals, after your 30-minute activity and during that activity. You can end your dinner with a small wedge of your wife's delicious cheesecake and/or a small scoop of that tasty "no sugar added" ice cream that you carefully chose after you read the label that day at the food store. Then you can gladly sit on your favorite couch and watch TV for the rest of the night.

So you see, the differences are not too drastic between the "asking for a massive heart attack and bring me all the diseases known to man" kind of lifestyle and the "I will make better lifestyle choices, better food choices and better activity choices during each and every day, and I will carefully indulge without feeling guilty and bring me loads of great health and send far away from me preventable and deadly diseases and their complications" kind of lifestyle. It is just a matter of choice. So which are you going to choose?

Remember, good health comes from small and flexible favorable habits that you pick up along the way of life and hold on to, which literally make a difference between life and premature death. If you think that you "messed up," then do better next time and keep going. For instance, if you forgot to do some walking or you didn't increase your activity during the day, it's okay, relax. Make a better choice next time, but don't give it up altogether; always remember that you are not on a diet and you are now making balanced choices. Get rid of the "perfection" mindset. It has nothing to do with your well-being.

The Common Actions of People Who Lost Weight And Kept It Off Permanently

After analyzing the patterns of people who lost weight and kept it off *permanently*, The National Weight Registry Agency has revealed the common habits of those who lost more than 30 pounds and kept them off for more than 3 years. The National Weight Registry Agency is an agency where anyone who lost more than 30 pounds and kept them off for more than 3 years can register.

Apply these steps now and watch your weight shed, as well as shedding the probability of acquiring those uninvited deadly diseases. Those who lose weight and keep it off employ the following steps and habits:

- They exhibit persistence.
- They remain constantly active during the day, and they schedule 30 minutes to an hour of sustained bouts of activity of their choice (walking, cycling indoors or outdoors, etc.) several days a week.
- They eat 3 main meals and 2 fruit snacks daily.
- They increase their intake of water.
- They reduce portion sizes of foods consumed.
- They eat and enjoy a balanced variety of food.
- They consume high-fiber food, eat fruits and vegetables several times per day, and consume little or no sugar or salty packaged foods and snacks.
- They adopt a balanced approach and avoid dieting (this means there is no failure).
- They weigh themselves frequently (once or twice a week).

Adopt these habits and start applying them now! Be in control of your weight, health and life!!!

The Process of Learning and Unlearning a Habit And How Any of Us Can Adapt

Every aspect of a human being, whether physical, mental or emotional, is adaptable. We can get into all kinds of good or bad habits depending on what we choose.

All of us can think of situations, which we had to adapt to regardless of how simple, or complex. For instance, think of a time when you owned a car where the parking brakes were activated by pressing with your left foot on the lower left pedal. Then you trade in your car for another where the parking brakes were activated by pulling with your right hand on a handle that is situated on the middle console between the driver and the passenger seats. As you drive your car initially, and you're trying to come to a full stop, and/or when you're trying to pull the parking brakes the first few times, you're going to try to erroneously push your left foot down in an effort to activate the parking brakes. But the parking brakes have changed location and they are no longer there. So you'll correct that action by pulling the brakes with your right hand to activate the parking brake. After persistent and repeated trials of activating the parking brake, you no longer habitually slam your left foot down in the wrong place, but you begin to activate it correctly with your right hand.

What has happened is that after several actions and persistent repetitions, you learned a new habit of pulling the parking brake with your right hand without hesitation, without making a conscious effort to locate the correct parking brake location. It just became second hand. You have also unlearned another habit, the habit of slamming your left foot down in order to activate the parking brake, which is now no longer there.

In essence, what you have done is that you have replaced the gap of the old habit with the new desired habit after repeated persistent actions and correct new actions that now form your new habit.

Likewise, any human being can learn new good habits, such as becoming more active and making better food choices and unlearn or drop the less favorable habits that are potentially dangerous to your health, such as: smoking, eating large portions of food, and selecting fattening and nutrient-deficient foods. All it takes is persistent repeated action to choose more favorable foods and snacks as in List A of the food section next, and after 3-4 weeks of daily and weekly such choices, you will develop better food selection habits with little effort to remember doing so. Actually, if you were trying to drop a bad habit such as smoking or snacking on fattening and nutrition-deficient food, the only way to fill the gap that this bad habit has created would be by replacing it with a favorable new habit.

Just remember the one crucial factor that successfully makes that new task a new habit; it is the initial 3-week concept; *expect* that you are going to mess up or forget to act on those new tasks. But you can correct the mix-ups during each following opportunity. Just keep on going and never give up. This is a normal and expected occurrence. Do not be hard on yourself. Perfection and rigid and inflexible expectations lead to failure. No one is or can become perfect. Just remember the new car with new parking brake location when you initially slammed your left foot down mistakenly to activate the parking brake, it was a minor inconvenience, and with persistent attempts at the correct action, you succeeded.

The Spandex Phenomenon

Yet, people who have been making the wrong food selections and have adapted to sitting in front of the tubes for hours on end daily and who lead sedentary lives and have been accumulating mega pounds for the last 40 or 50 years, expect to get up one Monday morning without prior preparation, go on a strict diet, with or without the help of over-the-counter diet pills, **get into a spandex outfit**, and start "exercising" for 2 hours a day. They pretend to know it all and with a "magic wand" or a "magic pill," fix it all in one week. "It ain't gonna happen." Of course things will not go their way, and with the first expected failure, they revert back to their old habits and back to packing on the pounds and piling on all the imaginable fatal dangers that can accompany obesity, sedentary lifestyles and out of control chronic diseases.

Build the Foundation First and Learn How to Fish

If you are trying to have lifelong good health or if you are trying to lose weight and keep it off permanently without establishing favorable patterns and lifestyle habits, it would be the same as me, who is trained as a pharmacist, one day deciding to build an Empire State Building double without consulting with engineers and architects, without a plan, and without financing; I embark on a task to build it myself. So I wake up one day and, without building a strong foundation to support a monument of that magnitude, I start piling up the bricks with cement and attempt to build my first wall. Am I going to get very far before that wall tumbles down? Certainly not.

Instead, lay the ground for building a strong foundation in order to build lifelong favorable lifestyle habits for lifelong good health, free of disease and/or of disease complications. If you have been overweight and sedentary, chances are you did not get there in a week or two, but rather it took you years and decades of faulty eating and snacking habits and inactivity habits. So, don't expect to reverse the situation in one week or two. Take the first 3 to 4 weeks on the journey of lifelong good health by establishing positive and healthy eating and activity lifestyle habits and patterns.

THE TRANSFORMATION INTO MORE FAVORABLE LIFESTYLE HABITS WILL REQUIRE YOU TO:

1. Take small persistent actions of practicing healthier food choices, including snacks; and remember to increase your activity daily and weekly.

2. If you forget or mess up, FORGIVE YOURSELF, don't be too harsh on yourself; make a better choice next time. Remember, if you aim at perfection, you will certainly fail, but aim at making favorable lifestyle choices most of the time (about 80% of the time). When you fall for that pizza, enjoy it, don't feel regret, because that would have fallen under the 20% not so favorable choices that you are ALLOWED, and the "I am proudly not so perfect" category. Your progress will not stop if you "mess up" 10% or 20% of the time. But your progress will stop if you "mess up" 80% of the time, and that's how people lose their battle with obesity and succumb to the deadly powers of disease complications.

3. Repeat actions daily and weekly. Three to four weeks later, you will have established some new habits and will be in the process of reaping the benefits for a lifetime, including losing weight and keeping it off permanently with your *persistent* favorable actions!

With your quest to make improved lifestyle choices during the initial 3-week period and even later, you must expect to "mess up" and occasionally forget to bring healthy snacks with you to work, or to take that extra walk; but after 3 weeks, you will remember from the first attempt to make the extra walking trips at work and at home, and you will remember to bring your snacks from home without forgetting (just like the parking break and all the examples I mentioned above). You will make better fast food meal choices at fast food and other type restaurants and you will be in control, juggle and balance all the variables. Even after that initial period of 3 weeks is up, you will keep on improving choices all the time. REMEMBER THAT THIS IS A PROCESS AND IN NO WAY RESEMBLES AN "ON AND OFF" SWITCH.

Never Feel Guilty Again

Never feel guilty again because you indulged occasionally, but attempt to do better next time and **remember that you can make not so favorable lifestyle choices 20% of the time and you will still achieve the health results you want, such as losing weight and keeping your sugar, cholesterol and blood pressure under control. People can achieve good health by making favorable lifestyle choices most of the time. One will not have bad health from missing an activity one day or one extra eating ice cream and a brownie one day a week.** The opposite is true. When you live like John Doe (see John Doe's story above), before he made lifestyle changes, every day of the week, then you will expect to suffer the grave and life-threatening consequences of bad health.

Do We Need Willpower to Have Good Health?
(MUST READ)

The saying, "One needs willpower to be able to lose weight, quit smoking, and to consequently have good health," is absolutely false. All you need is to make a habit of making favorable lifestyle choices in order to receive or to reap the rewarding and awesome benefits of good health.

Just remember to be persistent in your actions and practice moderation and balance in your choices by taking small steps at a time. **If you adopt moderation in your actions, you will be able to enjoy just about everything in life.** When you "mess up" forgive yourself, improve your choices next time, and keep going. When you aim at perfection you will fail. Practice moderation. Making favorable lifestyle choices in order to achieve good health must be every human being's mission and quest whether overweight or not or whether having disease or as a preventive measurement. *Without good health, life and the enjoyment of life cease to exist and are not worth living.*

Bye-Bye, Willpower—Hello Favorable Lifestyle Choices
Never, Ever Diet Again

Practice Positive Self-Talk, Visualization and the Power of Prayer

Positive Self-Talk

In the process of making more favorable lifestyle choices, pay attention as to how you talk to yourself and what messages you allow others to pass on to you. If you are one of those people who crack jokes about yourself, or send negative messages to yourself regarding your size or your inability to achieve a certain task, or if you allow others to talk that way about you, then don't. Your conscious and/or subconscious mind will believe anything it hears, and it makes whatever you hear (even jokingly) a firm reality. Instead, you need to say to yourself, "out loud" (a tone you can hear, not necessarily screaming) words that consist of positive messaging, several times daily and weekly. By doing so, you are unleashing a powerful tool, "your brain," to work in your favor. You can invent your own messages to say to yourself out loud; here are some examples:

- I feel good.
- I am worth it.
- I will lose the weight.
- I will make better food choices.
- I will become more active.
- I can quit smoking.
- I am a winner.
- I look great.
- Life is beautiful.
- I can make better lifestyle choices.
- (The list goes on.)

Visualization

Visualization is a powerful technique that boosts your effort to making a desired goal a reality. "See yourself" changed. *Form a mental picture of how you will feel and look* once that change takes place. For instance, if you are trying to make better food choices and you're trying to snack on fruits or mixed nuts instead of snacking on packaged snacks from the store such as peanut butter cookies or what you have handy, then take a couple of minutes during the day, close your eyes, and see yourself committing that action of actually seeing yourself in your mind's eye eating that broccoli and a vegetable dip; or visualize yourself making better food choices as you are ordering in a restaurant and see yourself chewing on healthier foods.

You can do the same regarding raising your level of activity during the day, by seeing yourself in your mind's eye doing that extra walking at work or while shopping. Visualize yourself making that extra loop to get to a certain item on the shelf. The more you practice, the better you get at it.

The Power of Prayer

Do not underestimate the power of prayer. Praying, according to your religious beliefs, can be an important factor and a contributor in helping you execute favorable actions in order to achieve your endeavor (of gaining and maintaining good health and warding off disease). Also praying can help you heal physically as well as spiritually and be at peace with God. This blessing peace can help bring you inner happiness regardless of your daily heavy load of stresses and burdens. In turn this internal happiness can be a powerful weapon in alleviating stress. When daily stress is reduced then blood sugar and blood pressure will follow suit and can bring diabetes into better control contributing to preventing diabetes complications. As a result of reducing the risk of complications you will have a better quality of life and you are even happier. Thus the body soul connection through the power of prayer is a strong link and you can seek it.

Making Balanced Food Choices

The Story of Toya Who Is Diabetic and Frustrated With "Low-Carb Diets"

A customer came up to the pharmacy consultation window where I was working one day and requested to speak to the pharmacist. When I came to the consultation window, I saw an attractive 55-year-old lady, Toya, who had gathered several over-the-counter weight-loss products and proceeded to ask me, in all frustration, which of them I recommended for weight loss and which of them would not interfere with her diabetes, blood pressure, and cholesterol medications.

Toya was overweight, had diabetes, high blood pressure, and high cholesterol. She told me she was fed up with trying diet after diet; the most recent being the "Low-Carb Diet" that everybody (and their mother) was on. "Every time I lose some weight, I gain it right back," she added. My first response was to discourage her from taking any of the over-the-counter diet pills that she brought me, not only because she had been taking her prescription medications, but because the long-term outcome of taking these diet pills is unknown and may contain herbs that may raise her blood pressure and worsen her blood pressure control. Moreover these "quick fixes" may be more harmful to her self-esteem than the failing diets she had become used to trying when she will regain the weight back.

I empathized with her frustration and anger and asked her to tell me more about her "Low-Carb Diet" and what exactly she was trying to achieve. She told me her goal was to be "thin"; she wanted to lose 60 pounds and have "6 packs abs" before her high school reunion in about 4-5 months. So she went on "that diet" a couple of months prior, and she had vowed to make it work this time. So she cut out bread, pasta, rice and desserts from her diet, all her favorite foods. She also joined the gym and had been "exercising" for about 1 to 1½ hours every day for at least 5 days a week. Additionally, during the weekend, she would go out for an hour walk each day. After 6 weeks of doing this, she had lost about 23 pounds and never felt any better. Her short-lived success boosted her self-esteem, and she was able to fit into clothing she had not been able to wear in years. She started receiving compliments about her new looks everywhere she went. She felt very proud of her achievement.

After a while, she started noticing strong cravings and felt that temptations were growing. Wherever she went, she would bump into bakeries and pastry shops with window displays loaded with eye-popping and mouth-watering decadent delights and sumptuous spreads of all kinds. She started dreaming of chocolate chip cookies, and the cravings only got stronger. One Friday night, she went out for dinner with her husband, and she ordered a long-awaited "half-pounder" bacon cheeseburger loaded with mayo and the bun was drenched with grease, along with a hearty order of French fries and an extra large soft drink. She finished off that evening with a large serving of double-fudge German-chocolate cake topped with whipped cream.

After completing that meal, she felt a short-lived sense of contentment coupled with feelings of regret and guilt. The next morning, she rushed to the bakery and ate two chocolate croissants for breakfast. Then she went on a spree (or what others call a binge) and indulged that whole weekend. Moreover, she had not been to the gym that whole week since it was taking too much of her time and piles of work at her job and at home were creeping up on her. The result of that weekend spree was that she gained 3 pounds and her sugar levels went up to an all-time high, and so did her blood pressure. Slowly, she reverted back to her old eating habits and stopped going to the gym and had regained all the weight she had lost plus two more pounds. In the process, she lost much self-esteem.

At this stage, as she was telling me all of this, her eyes watered. She finished her story by describing her disappointment in herself and told me how ugly she felt inside and out, and how depressed she felt for "failing big." I could feel exactly the pain Toya was going through as I had battled obesity myself, as I mentioned before, all through my childhood and adolescence until the age of 17. After being a dieting victim myself and having tried all the diets available, I had gone through the extremes of feeling proud when I would lose the weight to feeling morose and experiencing such a self-loathing sentiment, coupled with low self-esteem, as soon as I would regain the weight. I knew, firsthand, what she was going through.

I had acknowledged her sad feelings but rushed to congratulate her for taking action to do something about her weight. And I consoled her by making her aware that losing one battle does not mean losing the war. I emphasized to her that great success only comes after great failures. At least she was in the action phase and she attempted to find a solution to her problem. Countless others have more threatening and more severe lifestyle-related problems and are not even contemplating taking any action in the near future.

I also pointed out to her that she has great drive, and that all she needed were some modifications to her actions, and she could be well on her way to culling permanent satisfactory results. I also could not help but tell her, genuinely, that she looked beautiful, regardless of her current weight. At that point, I was able to notice a small smile forming on her face.

I wanted to find out from her, in her own words, what prevented her from moving forward with that "Low Carb Diet" and her loaded "exercise" program. She said, "It was restrictive, I just could not take it any longer. As for {exercise}, it took so much of my time and I got behind on every thing. I think my willpower is weak anymore."

I pointed out to her that she was not alone in this dilemma of "dieting," but that millions like her, including me, have gone through the disappointing journey of the "dieting game." Millions like her have been deceived and misled by all the "diet" programs that promise quick fixes and quick results, but what they don't tell you is how disappointed you will be when you see, before your eyes, how quickly your hard-earned efforts have evaporated as you regain your weight. What they also do not tell you is that the restrictive "diet" approach will *never* be a permanent solution for the weight dilemma and health epidemics that are threatening you and millions of others in this country. I also quickly pointed out to her that taking actions towards having good health and losing weight has nothing to do with her "willpower."

We, as a society, have been bombarded every hour of every day by messages from the media to become "thin," just like the lean male and female supermodels. I can assure you, Toya, that the definition of good health is not being thin or having "6 pack abs" like they depict on those commercials and on their supermodels. These models are professionals and spend several hours a day struggling to look the way they look. They are under constant pressure and scrutiny from their employers to keep their weight down, otherwise they could lose their jobs, and their weight is monitored daily. They are on strict diets that promote food deprivation and that lack essential nutrients. They live under constant pressure to stay thin, and by doing so; they lead highly stressful lives, which promote physical and mental illness. Those "look at me I look thin and great" models, in reality are not models of good health.

Lifelong good health is not a part-time job that starts on a Monday and ends on a Friday some weeks later. It can only be the result of favorable lifestyle habits and choices that can last a lifetime. Avoiding perfection (balance) and setting flexible and realistic goals, will take you several steps (and leaps) closer to your goal of achieving and maintaining lifelong good health. Making balanced food and activity choices daily is the only way you and anyone else can regain your dignity and control over your weight, your disease and your health. Having said that, your setting exaggerated and unrealistic goals, such as wanting to be "thin," losing 60 pounds, and having "6 pack abs" in four months (before your high school reunion) are the very same perfectionist goals that led you to fail.

Can you really see it in your mind's eye to be deprived of bread, rice, and pasta and your favorite desserts for life? How about tweaking your goals just a bit? Instead of aiming at "being thin," wouldn't it appeal more to you to aim at having a better self-image and a better quality of life? In the process you will lose weight as well. Does it seem more realistic and more achievable to you to be able to lose 1-2 pounds a week to a total weight loss goal of about 30 or 40 pounds that first year? I also suggested that she should not worry about her weight or looks for the high school reunion deadline because she looks great already.

When you start a "diet," Toya, at some point in time, you will have to end it, and with it, you will have to put a stop to your hard-earned results, as those will come to an end, too. It is only when you make balanced lifestyle choices that do not include deprivation or extreme actions, that you can maintain these habits over a lifetime.

The biggest mistake you can make is to deprive yourself of any food category. Your brain creates an internal balance by remembering any nutrient or food you have been exposed to throughout life. The main function of our brain is survival and to keep us alive. It does so by establishing and maintaining internal balances of all internal systems. Any deviation from that balance through a loss of any nutrient or food, regardless of whether you are trying to lose weight, or not, is construed by the brain as "an emergency situation."

The brain then will start a cascade of reactions in order to bring back that internal balance. Once that food becomes extinct from your diet, then your brain senses that big change and switches to the survival mode and thinks that you are in danger and consequently starts its reactions to re-establish that balance. It unleashes its fury by giving you craving signals to consume that "missing" food. The longer the period that this food is not detected in your body, the stronger those craving signals become. What you have unknowingly created is a situation in your brain called "rebound appetite" which can get you to even hallucinate and dream of that missing food until you give in and eat it, which explains your dreams about cookies. Except now, when you start eating this "missing" food, you do so with a vengeance by consuming large quantities; and by doing so, you will regain the weight you have worked so hard to lose. This explains what happened to you that infamous weekend when you had dinner out with your husband and ate gigantic portions of all the foods that you missed.

The only way you can achieve your realistic weight loss goals is to **not deprive** yourself from "any" food, including your favorite ethnic foods and desserts. Only, eat them in reduced portion sizes and proportionately balance all of the food groups.

I then gave Toya some food and snack suggestions that are balanced in nutrients, low in sugar, and high in fiber (See List A in the food section for a detailed list). I also gave her tips to increase her water consumption to about 6-8 glasses daily, and to switch from regular soda to diet soda or artificially sweetened iced tea. As for the activity, I told her, "You need to include a regimen that will not impose on your lifestyle but will blend right in with your lifestyle. So the gym can be wherever you want it to be." I gave her tips to increase the amount of walking she does at work, home and while shopping. I also told her to grab her husband and take him along for a brisk 30-45 minute walk about 3-4 times a week.

Now, Toya, do you think you could fit these activity tips in your daily lifestyle better than that 3-hour ordeal you had to experience every day in the gym? One thing you ought to remember when making lifestyle choices about food or activity is that you will not always make the best choices. When you don't make a very favorable choice, it's okay. Move along. You did not "blow your diet," just make a better choice next time and don't aim at perfection. When you occasionally indulge (and you should) then that falls in the remaining 20% of your off-task time. Never feel guilty again or put yourself down for not making a very good choice. Do the opposite. You need to **reward** yourself periodically. Again, "never" aim at perfection because if you do, you will certainly fail.

This is what making favorable lifestyle choice is all about? Just these small changes to Toya's lifestyle will get her to lose about 2 pounds a week, keep them off and regain her self-esteem, her dignity, and keep her diabetes and weight under control "permanently." Toya smiled and shook my hand with gratitude. I could feel that a heavy burden had been lifted off her shoulders.

Food Choices

Lose Weight and Keep It Off by Making Food Choices as Follows

The recommendations in the 80s and 90s to raise the consumption of "carbohydrates" and to reduce drastically the consumption of "fat" since fat has almost single handedly been blamed for the obesity epidemic in the USA. The net result was the reverse of what was expected and obesity has tripled since then (refer to the "Obesity statistics" on page 122 around the beginning of Action Step 4). It was not difficult to figure out the reasons. People went on a rampage of consuming "mega" portions of white breads, white rice and white pasta and "Fat Free" packaged snacks of cookies, chips containing nothing but mega calories of refined sugar, fat and salt.

Eating such foods high in sugar content causes a sharp rise in blood sugar levels causing insulin to rise sharply as well (as is discussed in detail in the next paragraph titled "Carbohydrates"). The presence of high amounts of insulin in the blood causes weight gain, raises the blood pressure and blood cholesterol which all can drastically increase the chances of heart disease, heart attacks and strokes.

As a result to the failing "high sugar diets" the response came in the late 90s by tipping the balance to the opposite end and blaming the "Carbs" for all our health problems including the rise in obesity and the rising incidence of chronic diseases such as diabetes, high blood pressure, high cholesterol, heart and artery disease. This has lead to the rise of "Protein Diets." Those diets promoted the elimination from meals of almost all of the "Carbs" including fruits at least in the initial few weeks while allowing the consumption of enormous amounts of foods containing fats and proteins. That did not solve the problem either because of these and any other "Diets" restrictive nature and for other reasons discussed in detail in the section about "Protein Diets" and their health consequences a couple paragraphs down).

The solution is balancing the proportions of the various food groups and portion sizes and doing away with "diets" and the "diet" mind set. Also making food or carbohydrate choices that are higher in fiber content from List A has all the benefits of preventing disease reducing hunger, reducing the sugar and cholesterol in the blood and promoting permanent weight loss. So instead of choosing the white version of bread how about all the other delicious whole grain, rye, sourdough or pumpernickel versions. Instead of the white version of rice how about the brown or Basmati kind. Instead of white pasta how about the whole-wheat version of it. Similar substitution to the healthier versions of all other food categories along with reducing portion sizes is at the heart of food choices and recommendations in this guide. That is what we will discuss in detail next.

The playing field has leveled off between the dietary recommendations for those who have diabetes and for those who don't. For ultimate disease and disease complications prevention, weight control and loss, end of the hunger cycle and the end to the yoyo results, reduce (not cut out) the sugar consumption, raise fiber intake and balance other foods choices and portion sizes as follows:

- Carbohydrates 50-55%
- Fat 25-30%
- Protein 20-25%

What does this all mean and how is it practically achieved in terms of making daily food choices? First, let's find out what each of these building blocks of life (nutrients) called carbohydrates, fats, and proteins are all about.

All foods available to humans belong to either one or more of these three major food categories: carbohydrates, fats, and proteins. The main function of food is to provide energy to various body and muscle functions in order to sustain life. Each of these categories is equally essential to life in different and complementary ways. Consuming food in a balanced manner (as in the proportions mentioned above) is essential and promotes good health and wards off diseases and their complications.

However, these same foods, when consumed in excess, promote weight gain and bring us deadly diseases.

What Are Carbohydrates?

Foods belonging to this category provide humans with the primary source of energy in the form of glucose, or in common terms, glucose is known as sugar. When common foods such as bread, pasta, rice, cereal and potatoes are consumed, they pass through the intestines and, in the process, get broken down into their final form as glucose or sugar. This sugar passes from the intestines to the blood stream via a web of blood vessels connected to the intestines. As we eat more of these carbohydrate foods, sugar continues to rise in the blood stream. When it exceeds a baseline of 100 points (mg/dl), then your brain signals a hormone named insulin to be released from your pancreas to your blood stream to help store that excess sugar into your liver and all your body muscles in the form of a substance called **glycogen** (as discussed in the insulin section in Action Step 2). The glycogen that is now stored in your muscles and liver will be used at a later stage when your body calls on it as an initial energy source for short-movement tasks such as getting up from your chair to the kitchen to get water.

UNLOCKING THE PUZZLE OF HOW THE EXCESS SUGAR AND FOOD YOU EAT ENDS UP AS FAT UNDER YOUR SKIN

Say it's time to clean house, and you want to empty the trash from 3 different locations in your 2-story house. Say you want to try to increase the amount of activity you do and you make 3 different trips from each of these 3 trash can sites to the dumpster outside your house. Each round trip from the trash site to the dumpster takes about 2-3 minutes, and each bag weighs about 2-3 pounds. Although this seems an easy task, it actually requires a lot of sophisticated, coordinated movements from the leg, arms and mid-section body muscles, requiring energy. Where did this instant energy for the short 2-3 minute bout of movement come from? It came from the sugar that's in your blood and the sugar that has been stored in your muscles and liver called glycogen.

On your first trip to the dumpster, you may have used some of the sugar that is readily available in your blood. And for the subsequent trips, you have consumed some of that glycogen that has been stored in your liver and muscles. This glycogen, once again, breaks down to sugar, which is glucose, and is consequently used as an immediate source of energy to fuel your working muscles. This sugar that has been used up in this situation gets replenished from the next snack or meal you will consume.

What happens if you are a sedentary person and do not perform the action of disposing of the trash but delegate it to someone else? Then you would not have used up that sugar from your muscles. Moreover, what if you have not been making favorable food selections and you have been eating, excessively, foods from a typical "Western Diet" such as super-sized burger combos, including a large soda, or a pizza. Then you have bread, fries and 16-ounce regular soft drink all belonging to the sugar family named "carbohydrates." All of these foods will break down in your body to their final form (glucose or sugar).

Since you ate so much from the same food groups, you're going to have a lot of sugar dumped into your blood stream. And since you have not been active and you didn't pick up the trash yourself, the sugar already stored in your muscles and liver has not been used up and is saturated in those sites. What is your body going to do with all the excess sugar you just consumed? This excess sugar will have no place else to go but to be converted to fat which will then be stored under your skin. As you keep repeating the cycle of inactivity and excessive eating, more fat gets accumulated under your skin; that is how you gain weight.

This excess of fat also causes a rise in cholesterol and increases the risk of heart disease. Any food consumed in excess ends up contributing to:

- Weight gain
- A rise in cholesterol
- A rise in blood pressure
- A rise in the risk of heart disease

However, when making balanced food choices, you can lose weight and, at the same time, enjoy your favorite **great-tasting** food.

In any food category, the kinds and amounts of food you train yourself to eat make a whole lot of difference. This can be a major factor in determining whether you gain or lose weight, whether you have good or bad health, whether you are constantly threatened with disease, and whether you control your diabetes or not. The amount of sugar contained in food determines how much glucose or sugar will be dumped into the blood after consumption.

Glycemic Index

The amount of sugar that is contained in food and consequently becomes available in your blood stream is referred to as the Glycemic Index of that food, and it is a percentage. The higher the amount of sugar in foods or the higher the Glycemic Index, such as white bread and white rice, the easier it is to transform that food into fat when consumed, and the less fiber and nutritive value it contains. Carbohydrates are divided into two groups: simple and complex carbohydrates.

Carb Counting

"Carb counting" can be an important tool for all diabetics to help bring their blood sugar under controls especially those on intensive insulin therapy or on an insulin pump. You will need to inject 1 unit of short acting insulin such as Humalog, Novolog, Humulin or Novolin R for every 15 gm of Carbs you will be consuming at that meal.

The following foods and portions are examples of a serving, which includes 15gm of Carbs:

- One slice of whole grain bread
- 1 small baked potato with skin
- Brown rice, mashed potatoes or brown pasta (enough to fill a quarter of an average size round plate)
- 1 medium-size fruit
- One scoop of ice cream (If you will be consuming a sugar free ice cream then you do not count it)
- 1 biscuit

If you plan to have a salad (without croutons), brown rice, a grilled chicken breast and one slice of whole grain bread then finish your lunch with one medium scoop of ice cream. Prior to that lunch you will need to inject 3 units of short action insulin. Use one unit for the brown rice, one unit for the one slice of whole grain bread and one unit for the ice cream. Remember to test your sugar first before any insulin injection (as indicated in Action Step 3) and use the proper insulin injection technique (as indicated in Action Step 2).

Simple Carbs

"**Simple Carbs" have high sugar contents** or a high Glycemic Index up to 100%. Foods in this group have the least amount of fiber in them, if at all, and cause a quick rise in blood sugar, a quick rise in insulin, and they consequently **cause hunger within a short period of time after their consumption. They have the least nutritive value, are less filling, and greatly contribute to weight gain and diseases.** Generally, the more processed the food, the less fiber and the less nutritive value it contains "and" the higher its contribution to weight gain.

For example, one slice of white bread, which is completely stripped of fiber (0.5 grams or less fiber per slice) and nutrients will have 100% sugar content as it reaches your blood, and it will make you hungry in about 30 minutes or so. Whereas, its whole grain (Complex Carbs) counterpart or pumpernickel bread of the same size, will have a whopping 50% less sugar content once it hits your blood stream "and" will also have a lot of fiber (up to 4 or 5 grams per slice which ten-fold more than white bread) and a number of nutrients and vitamins.

Examples of processed foods are:
- White bread
- White pasta
- White rice
- All high sugar, fat and salty packaged snacks

For a detailed list of foods containing refined sugar, please refer to the extensive list of foods belonging to the various food groups further down in this section. (This does not mean that you should cut these foods out completely; just eat them less frequently, say a couple of times per week, and in smaller portions. The rest of the weekdays make the higher fiber selections. (Remember the 80% better choices and 20% less favorable choices we have extensively discussed already!)

BREAKING THE HUNGER CYCLE "CODE"

In the beginning of the section "What Are Carbohydrates?" I was telling the story of the journey that sugar makes from the time it is in that glazed donut or slice of white bread until it gets broken down in your gut/digestive system and then passes through to your blood. I also mentioned that as the sugar level rises above 100 points in the blood, it triggers insulin to be secreted from your pancreas. Well, when you make a food choice from the simple sugars or a food choice that has a high Glycemic Index (meaning food that is "very" high in sugar such as: candy, white bread, or others in this category; see List B further down for a detailed list of high sugar containing food) then this causes a very high and quick amount of insulin to be released into your blood.

When this happens, insulin lowers the amount of sugar in your blood aggressively and quickly to as low as below 100 points because that is how your pancreas reacts to foods with high sugar content. When your sugar drops below 100 points, it automatically sends a signal to your brain that you are hungry; remember, your brain's main function is to keep you alive and to keep everything "normal" and at a balance and a blood sugar balance that your brain registers is 100 points (mg/dl), and any deviation from that balance triggers an emergency response from your brain to correct that deviation from the norm.

The brain does not really care that you are dieting or snacking but is only concerned about your "survival," all must be level and normal in your body, according to your brain. In this case, within 20-30 minutes of consuming that high-sugar snack, you will feel hunger and the need to eat again. Not only this, but also if you refer to the insulin section in Action Step 2, we discussed that insulin's main function is not only to move excess sugar from your blood and store it in your liver and muscles, but another function is to also efficiently store fat from the food you eat into the fat storage sites under your skin.

So when you go on an eating spree or binge, eating high volumes of food containing sugar and fat, you cause insulin to be secreted in high amounts, and it not only helps reduce sugar from your blood but insulin also efficiently stores fat. In addition, what happens to all the excess sugar you eat? Since you have been inactive, sugar has not been used up from your muscles and the sugar stores there are full and saturated and the only fate that excess sugar will have is to be transformed into "fat." DOUBLE WHAMMY. Remember, the more sugar a food contains (refer to List B of less favorable food options next), the higher the Glycemic Index, the lower the fiber, and the higher the insulin response, as well as the heightened hunger factor and the potential to eat more and more (Catch 22).

SOLUTION: Make food choices, most of the time, from the Complex Carbs (for the reasons discussed in the next paragraph) and all the other food groups (See List A, next, for an extensive list of favorable choices from all food groups). Choose foods less frequently from the Simple Carbs and from the less favorable food choices (in List B).

Complex / High Fiber Carbs (A Better Choice)

High Fiber Carbs break down slowly in your body and do not trigger high sugar peaks and, consequently, trigger a lower insulin response, and a much delayed hunger response. Complex Carbs food also provides you with steady energy for your working muscles throughout the day and they are crucial sources of vitamins especially vitamins B-Complex and folates (B-complex and folates protect you from heart disease and they are necessary elements in aiding in the digestion of food) that are necessary for life. Although they may have much less of a tendency to be transformed into fat when consumed in balanced amounts, if they are consumed in very large quantities, they can also contribute to weight gain, just like any other food when consumed in excessive portions.

Examples of high fiber or Complex Carb foods are (See "Carbs" in List A for an extensive list further down):

- Whole grain bread
- Oat bran
- Oats
- All bean products
- Lentils
- Peas
- Vegetables
- Fruits

Whole grain breads or high fiber food will not make you hungry and can hold you for several hours because they break down slowly in your body and cause very little insulin to be released from your pancreas.

A Word about Beans

Beans, lentils and peas in all their forms, have been shown to carry amazing health and heart protective benefits. They are a major source of fiber, Complex Carbs, proteins, vitamins and folates. **Studies have shown when people consume beans four or more times weekly, their diabetes is in better control and the risk of heart disease is considerably less.** Cook them any way you'd like, but try to skip or reduce the amount sugar in some bean preparations such as "Baked Beans." Eat in less frequency the Mexican style refried beans as they may contain Lard (pork fat). For a more extensive list of foods high in fiber and low in sugar, refer to List A in "The Meal Blueprint" section later on in this Action Step 4.

Lifestyle Choices

PROVEN BENEFITS OF SELECTING FOODS HIGH IN FIBER AND LOW IN SUGAR:

- Stops the hunger cycle.
- Creates weight loss of up to a half pound per week (**if you consume 35gm of fiber daily, you burn an additional 250 calories per day**).
- Aids in long-term weight control.
- Can prevent or reverse heart disease.
- Helps you burn more fat at rest.
- reduces stroke risk.
- Decreases cholesterol and triglyceride in the blood.
- Decreases fat absorption from the food you eat.
- Decreases sugar absorption from the food you eat.
- If you already have diabetes, consuming food that is higher in fiber content and lower in sugar along with activity helps you keep the fasting sugar levels below the recommended 110 mg/dl, brings diabetes under control and reduces the exhaustion to the pancreas' capacity to produce insulin. This eventually may delay the need to use insulin later on.
- Helps you prevent diabetes complications.
- If you don't have type 2 diabetes but are predisposed to getting it (see detailed criteria in Action Step 1), consuming foods that are high in fiber and lower in sugar along with an active lifestyle, will help you prevent acquiring diabetes by making your pancreas get less exhausted in producing excess insulin.
- Makes you feel full.
- Keeps your bowels regular by its bulking effect (when drinking 6 to 8 glasses of water daily).
- Reduces the risk of colon cancer.

The daily fiber recomendations for good health is 35 grams.

HOW TO GET 35 GRAMS OF FIBER DAILY AND LOSE AN ADDITIONAL 250 CALORIES DAILY

Currently most people are consuming on average about 10 to 14 grams of fiber daily. Remember that by increasing, **alone**, your daily fiber intake to about 35gm you will burn an additional 250 calories daily and you will get all the health benefits from fiber as discussed above. This is **easily done**. The high fiber cereals (from the "High Fiber Carbs,"

"Breakfast Choices" section in List A) can provide you with up to 14 grams of fiber (per serving as mentioned on the cereal's Nutrition Label). For lunch and dinner when you eat high fiber carbs such as beans, brown rice or pasta enough to cover a quarter of that round plate or 2 slices of whole grain bread, (see more choices for high fiber carbs in List A) that will get you 8 to 10 grams of fiber for each meals. Add on top of that 5 to 10 grams of fiber daily that you will get from the veggies and the fruits and you will be well over 35 grams of fiber daily. Please keep in mind that by raising your daily fiber consumption, you are not only getting the benefit of expanding an additional 250 calories and further weight loss benefits but also loads of other benefits as discussed above.

Try This at Home to Visually Witness the Impact That Foods with High or Low Sugar Content Have on Your Blood Sugar Levels

As a diabetic, a visual motivator would be for you to test your blood sugar with your blood sugar monitor about 45 minutes to an hour after a high-fiber meal containing any type of beans or whole grain vs. a typical cheeseburger combo with fries, a large regular soft drink and cookies. See, first-hand, the eye-popping spikes in blood sugar that take place if you opt for the high sugar, high fat meal. Even if you are not diabetic and have access to a blood sugar monitor you need to try this.

Water Consumption and Fiber

When making high-fiber food choices, it is imperative that you drink about 8 glasses of water per day. The bulking effect and the benefits of fiber require water consumption.

Sugar Alcohols as Sweeteners:

They include:
- Sorbitol
- Maltitol
- Galactitol
- Mannitol
- Xylitol
- Erythritol
- Isomol

These are carbohydrates that are not completely broken down in the body and consequently minimally impact your blood sugar. About 50% of sugar alcohols get slowly absorbed into the blood so having a snack containing no more than 3 or 5 grams of sugar alcohol is appropriate. Food manufacturers use them as sweetening agents in products such as chocolate bars, low-carb and energy bars. They are safe for consumption by people with diabetes. However, some people may have low stomach tolerance for them, as they may causes bloating and/or diarrhea. Watch your consumption of various snacks containing these agents, as this may worsen the stomach side effects. Read nutrition labels of foods you eat.

Sweeteners

All sweeteners available in the market nowadays are safe for human consumption and can assist people in lowering their dependence on sugar when used in daily balanced amounts to sweeten foods and drinks. Splenda is one of the highest quality sweeteners, as it has an identical texture to sugar, it tastes exactly like sugar, and you can use it for cooking and baking purposes; it also has no aftertaste and contains zero calories. Splenda does not contain Phenylalanine (see Warning about Phenylketoneurea next).

And by the way, as per a recent national consensus, all diet sodas and all sweeteners found in various foods and drinks are all absolutely safe for human consumption when consumed in balanced amounts daily.

Warning: However, having said that, there is a **contraindication and clear warning** for some people who have a condition named Phenylketoneurea. This is a **rare genetic** condition that is inherited and causes mental and physical retardation of the baby if not diagnosed and treated shortly after birth.

For the curious only: Phenylketoneurea is a result of a build up in the blood of a substance called Phenylalanine, which is an Amino Acid that is found in food substances that are protein such as meats, milk, eggs, grains, beans and other vegetables. Also, Aspartame containing sweeteners, after consumption, break down to produce Phenylalanine. People who have this disorder do not have the enzyme that breaks down Phenylalanine to another substance called Tyrosine resulting in the toxic buildup of Phenylalanine in the blood. If you do not know whether you have this condition then you don't. Babies who have this disorder cannot survive past the first few weeks or months of life without being treated accordingly otherwise mental and physical retardation or death may ensue. The FDA requires manufacturers to list in their Nutrition Labels whether any of their products contain Phenylalanine. **So read nutrition labels of foods you eat.** All people, young and old, who have this disorder, must **avoid** consuming Aspartame containing products. Likewise, women who are pregnant may not know whether their fetuses have this disorder and must get clearance from their gynecologists before consuming products containing Aspartame. Products like Splenda are a better substitute. If in doubt call your doctor.

"Net Carb" Count

The "Net Carb" term that you find on many food labels nowadays, is the amount of sugar that reaches your blood stream after the amount of fiber and sugar alcohols have been deducted. Let's take an example. Let's say you chose a dark chocolate bar or a cookie snack where "3 gm Net Carbs" was imprinted on that package. So you flip that snack to the nutrition label and start reading the content. Look at the " Total Carbohydrates" line and you might find "18g." The very next line may have "Dietary fiber 4g," the next line "Sugars 3g" and the next line will have "Sugar Alcohols 11g" (in other snacks or food labels sugar alcohols may be listed under "Other carbohydrates." If you do the math of all the last 3 figures you will get a total of 18 grams of Carbohydrates, however, of those 18gm only the 3 grams of sugar will reach your blood initially since fiber is minimally absorbed. However, keep in mind that as is mentioned in the "Sugar Alcohols" section, sugar alcohols will be breakdown slowly and eventually about 50% reach your blood but some manufacturers list the "Net Carbs" without accounting for 50% of Carbs from sugar alcohols. **Become a label reader of the food you eat.**

Hence the "Net Carb" in that snack is equal to 3 grams plus the 5grams that will be absorbed from sugar alcohols at a later stage. What you want to also look for in that snack is balanced amounts of fats and proteins as well. In a 100 calorie snack 2 to 3 grams of fat and 4 to 6 grams of proteins may be adequate for that snack. Moreover, watch for those 11 grams of sugar alcohol since they may cause stomach discomfort, bloating, flatulence and diarrhea. The lesser the amount of sugar alcohols the lesser the discomfort. **Other snacks may be sweetened with Splenda instead of sugar alcohols while preserving the taste of sugar.**

Deciphering "Low Carb Diets"

First, the word "diet" gives it away. A "diet" is always restrictive of some foods, and one cannot maintain "a diet" permanently; a "diet" is a temporary state. The authors of these Low Carb Diets recommend the restriction of all carbs including fruits in the "initial phases" of the diet. Reason being, when you cut out all forms of carbohydrates, then the sugar stores in your muscles and livers will get depleted. Remember the story about picking up trash and what we said about the first source of fuel when you perform a brief bout of activity. Your body will call on that first source of fuel, which is the sugar that has been stored in your muscles and your liver called Glycogen (see discussion in the " What are the Carbohydrates" section above). Once carb-depletion occurs after two weeks of cutting out carbohydrates from your meals, your body will start calling on the fat stores and start converting the fat into a substitute energy form called Ketones. Then you are in a state called "Ketosis." Ketones can be detected in the urine by performing a simple test that you buy over-the-counter called "Ketostix"

As a pharmacist, several times a week, I have customers ask me for urine Ketone strips, and I immediately know what they need them for. I realize that some diabetics may need to test periodically for the presence of "Ketones" in their urine for other purposes than dieting, but low carb dieters want to find out if "Ketones" are present in their urine which signals that their carbohydrates stores are already depleted. I proceed to tell them the consequences of the ketosis state.

First, Ketones are not efficient sources of energy and cannot provide your working muscles and brain with efficient fuel. Whenever you are in the state of fuel deprivation, your body will start breaking down your own muscles in order to be converted to sugar and consequently provide you with energy (you don't have to remember this; but this state is referred to pharmacologically as Gluconeogenesis). The net result of Ketosis type "Diet" is that you lose a good chunk of precious muscle mass. Also, whenever you lose your sugar stores (Glycogen), you also start losing water through urination to a total 4 pounds of precious water loss; and of course you lose some fat. **Since muscle weighs more than fat**, when it is lost for "dieting" purposes in the manner described here, it tips the weight scale further south. People on a diet feel good and get excited when they see their weight drop quickly initially but soon this quick weight loss stops. Loss of muscle mass causes the metabolic rate to drop and consequently fat weight regain becomes very likely. (See the discussion about the metabolic rate in detail in the activity section).

Not only that, but your brain's main fuel is glucose or sugar. Once your body glucose is depleted, your mental acuteness and memory suffers. Also, side effects of this diet, such as headaches, hair loss, and constipation, start affecting your quality of life. You also feel tired, due to loss of sodium and potassium because of dehydration, and you are less likely to remain active. You also have increased your chances of developing kidney stones and light headaches (which are due to reduced blood pressure). So Go through that whole ordeal of deprivation and compromised quality of life and these unpleasant side effects for weeks to do what? To activate your fat stores and lose weight?!!

Guess What Activates Your Body's Fat Stores in Just 4-5 Minutes And Helps You Burn Your Fat as Fuel and Consequently to Lose Weight and Keep It Off?

Regular Activity!

Read more about the magic of the benefits of activity to our health and to improving our quality of lives and ward off diseases and disease complications in the Activity Section subsequent to this section.

Fats

This building block of life has had a bad reputation during the '80s and '90s and has been unjustly accused of being responsible for the looming obesity crisis then. There was a "nationwide misleading recommendation" that urged us to cut down, drastically, fat consumption and that urged us to raise, to a major extent, the consumption of carbs such as: bread, rice, pasta and potatoes, without regard to their fiber content. All kinds of literature and books flooded the market promoting high carbs and very low-fat diets, blaming "fat" for all our health crises.

The food industry responded with the mega-production of processed foods and packaged candy, cookies, saltine snacks, salad dressings and countless other products labeled "Fat Free"; this indirectly or directly signaled people, misleadingly, that they could indulge in these foods and still lose weight, as long as they cut out the fat. People responded by reducing drastically their daily fat intake to as low as 10% of total daily food consumed and raising their carb intake sharply up to 70% or more of their total daily food consumed. Everyone started consuming mega snacks labeled "Fat Free."

This was very misguided and resulted in a health crisis of catastrophic proportions. Within 20 years, obesity had tripled and has now risen to up to 60% of the American population who suffer from being overweight or obese. Diabetes hit an all-time high and has now reached epidemic proportions, and there's no relief in sight for the next decade or two unless people start doing something about it **NOW.**

How Important Is "Fat" to Our Bodies?

Fat plays a vital role in our lives. Fat makes food taste better; in the past, using excessive amounts of fat was a sign of generosity and hospitality. Balanced amounts of fat promote fullness during and after a meal.

It is crucially important and necessary to consume good types of fat from the oils, nuts and fish kingdoms, especially those containing Omega-3 (see detailed lists of Omega-3 and beneficial sources of fats in "Fats and oils" and "Snacks section" in List A). Foods with beneficial sources of Fats and oils are also an important source of Vitamin E, which is an antioxidant. Foods such as olives, olive oil, mixed nuts, salmon, and many other fish products need to be consumed up to 4-5 times per week or more for their much valued health benefits. These foods and their nutrients are not only essential for good health, but they also promote cholesterol reduction and blood thinning, and they consequently protect the heart and arteries, preventing heart attacks and strokes. Of course, like any foods, when consumed in excess, they can promote weight gain, and their benefits will be reversed.

Fat, in the human body, serves several vital purposes. Among them is that fat, stored under our skin, cushions our precious internal organs and protects them from trauma and severe impact. Hair and skin all thrive and require a fatty medium. All our hormones bathe in an environment of fat. Vitamins A, D, E and K are stored in our body fat. Women need more fat in their bodies than men and consequently their dietary fat needs are slightly more than those of men. Women have more scalp hair than men and their skin is softer than men's; women's hormones are responsible for their monthly cycles, their pregnancies and deliveries. All of these situations make women require a healthy balance of fat in their bodies. Refer to List A for an extensive list of health friendly fat choices and portion sizes.

Consuming too little fat especially the beneficial Omega-3 foods and oils can have health consequences such as:

- Hair falling out
- Dry skin
- Shortage of vitamins (especially A, D, E and K)
- Increased PMS
- Trouble during menstrual cycles such as lack of or irregular cycles
- Loss of heart protective properties

On the other hand, consuming excessive amounts of "good fat" from favorable sources can lead to obesity, heart disease (the number one killer in women and men), and diabetes and will fuel diabetes complications and other deadly ailments. As for all food consumed a **key word here is Balance.**

The most important function that fat plays in our bodies is providing us and our working muscles with the largest source of energy. After 4-5 minutes of steady activity such as walking, cycling, swimming, playing sports, etc., which involve large muscle groups (such as the legs), fat storage sites under our skin are activated and called upon to break down and supply the working muscles with large sources of fuel until that steady activity is completed.

So the energy that our body needs during the first 3-4 minutes of any physical movement we make is derived from the sugar stores in the liver and muscles known as Glycogen. In the event that the activity were to continue past 3 or 4 minutes, then the energy required becomes greater, and the fuel gradually starts shifting from the sugar stores to the fat stores. So, it makes sense then to increase our level of activity throughout the day so we can burn more fat and lose more weight.

Good Fats (Unsaturated) vs. Bad Fats and Cholesterol (Saturated Fats)!

Good Fats (Unsaturated)

Some of foods containing "good" kinds of fats and Omega-3 fats (referred to as Unsaturated fats) are:

- Olive oil
- Canola oil
- Safflower and sunflower oils
- Nuts
- Seeds
- Avocados
- Olives
- Salmon
- Mackerel
- Tuna
- Herring (see List A for extensive list)

All of the above are major sources of good sources of fat and can lower cholesterol and the incidence of heart disease if consumed in balanced amounts. They can aid the body in ridding itself of "bad" cholesterol, which deposits itself around the arteries, eliminating it through the bowels.

Lifestyle Choices

Bad Fats and Cholesterol (Saturated)

Our body, namely our liver, produces 85% of the cholesterol we need. With the exclusion of palm and coconut oils, cholesterol from outside the body comes exclusively from animal sources. These food sources contain cholesterol and bad fats referred to as saturated fats such as:

- Fatty cuts of steak
- Fatty cuts of pork
- Fatty chicken skin
- Bacon
- Sausage
- Pepperoni
- Packaged snacks and foods containing "Trans Fatty Acid"
- Solid cooking fats (margarine/butter/lard) (see List B for an extensive list of these less favorable fats which need to be consumed less frequently, no more than once or twice a week)

Once these less favorable fats are consumed more frequently, they contribute to fat build-up around the arteries that lead to the heart and brain.

As portion sizes of typical western meals keep on getting bigger, it is not hard to saturate the remaining 15% of your cholesterol intake. The excess of these bad cholesterols and saturated fats will either linger in the blood, causing a rise in blood cholesterol; or they will be deposited, progressively over a period of time, around the arterial walls, restricting the flow of blood coming to the heart and brain by forming hardened layers of fat referred to as "Plaque."

At unknown times, this "Plaque" will rupture; and plaque fragments will completely block the flow of blood to either your heart or brain, causing a heart attack or a stroke. Plaque can be prevented from forming around the artery walls through the consumption of whole grain foods (foods high in fiber reduce the absorption of bad cholesterol and fats from the blood) and the good fats in balanced amounts along with regular daily activity (regular daily activity reduces the incidence of rising blood cholesterol and the consequent formation to plaque) and/or with the use of cholesterol-lowering drugs.

What You Should Remember From the Fat Section Of This Guide:

- Fats are not all bad; some are essential for life.
- Make food selections daily and in small portion sizes from favorable fat sources (see List A and meal plan for details): olive oil, nuts, seeds and fish as they have been shown to protect your heart from disease.
- Limit food selections from the bad fats; consume them only occasionally and, if possible, switch to heart-protective good fats 80% of the time.
- When eaten in excess, fats will make you gain fat pounds and consequently increase the risk of heart disease.

Proteins

Foods belonging to this last building block of life provide the body with nutrients necessary to perform vital functions. When proteins from lean meats (a considerable source of iron), pork, poultry, fish, beans and soy (see List A for an extensive list) are consumed, they break down in the intestines and get absorbed into the bloodstream as a final protein form called Amino Acids. Meats, pork, poultry and fish contain the highest amount of protein of all other food groups. Protein's main function in the body is tissue repair (which might be caused by trauma, a burn, or a workout). Proteins also play an essential role in metabolizing the food we eat through large protein molecules called enzymes. Without these enzymes, it would be impossible to digest food. Also, all hormones within the human body are made, in part, of protein.

Protein is the last energy source in our bodies and must not be used or depended upon to provide the body with energy. When the body uses protein as fuel, the person is either in "starvation mode," "under physical stress," or "on a diet" such as the "Low Carb Diet."

All of us have seen the heart-wrenching sight of people who are, literally, skin and bones, such as starving children in various countries especially in the African continent. In this case, their bodies have first consumed all the sugar stores until those stores were depleted; next, the fat stores were consumed until those stores were depleted, and they are the largest fuel source in the body. When no food is consumed, the muscles start breaking down to sugar in order to provide much needed fuel for survival. When this last phase occurs, it may be irreversible, even if food is consumed; often, these children eventually perish.

Another quick way to lose muscle is when you lose weight rapidly during a "diet," especially the Low-Carb diets. Refer to the discussion titled Deciphering "Low Carb Diets" for further details on this issue. Any time you are on a diet that restricts drastically the total number of daily calories and/or the consumption of carbohydrates, your brain calls on your muscle mass to breakdown some muscle cells and transform them to Glucose (or sugar), which is the body's first fuel source in order to replenish that energy gap.

WHAT YOU SHOULD REMEMBER FROM THE PROTEIN SECTION:

- Many non-meat food categories such as beans, lentils, peas, all the bean family and soy are all rich sources of protein.
- Lean protein sources such as meat, fish, pork, chicken, the bean family, dairy and soy are essential for survival and help our body recover from trauma, injury and exercise. Also, these foods help our digestive systems produce hormones and enzymes that are key and indispensable to food digestion, and are also muscle builders.
- When eaten in excess, proteins can cause weight gain, raise cholesterol, and cause kidney problems.

Become a Nutrition Label Reader

Read labels! Look for foods that have balanced amounts of nutrients. Such balanced foods or snacks, per serving amount indicated on that chosen food's Nutrition Label, are low in total calories (about 150 calorie), low in total Carbs (about 20 grams) with a reduced sugar content (less than 7 or 8 grams), high in fiber content (5 to 10 grams or more), balanced in fat content (about 4 to 5 grams) and **void of Trans Fats; and** balanced in protein content (about 5 to 7 grams). Don't just focus on one component of that Nutrition Label but look at the overall food distribution balance. Look for the overall calorie content and nutrient distribution as discussed above. Here's an example: you're trying to select a mid-afternoon dessert snack after you have consumed your fruit, and you select a marble cake. You are reading the label of that prepackaged marble cake, and you see that the total amount of calories for that one piece is 500. Of those, you have about 31 grams of fat calories, 40 grams coming from the sugars group (carbohydrates), with only about 4 grams coming from protein and only 1 gram coming from fiber.

Obviously, this would not be a favorable every day choice. However, a favorable choice would be two small squares of a dark chocolate bar because the portion size is more balanced and dark chocolate, in balanced amounts, has shown to have antioxidant and heart protective properties like Green Tea infusions. Moreover, dark chocolate has a lower content of sugar and a higher content of fiber in comparison to milk chocolate and other sugar laden chocolate bars. This and other favorable dessert choices from List A can be daily sources of "sweet snacks" if consumed in balanced amounts. Occasionally, you may desire to have an ice cream or a balanced portion of marble cake (or other dessert choices from List B) and you should. You are still in balance if you consume them less frequently, about once or twice a week, in balanced portion sizes. You should throw guilt out the window since you were making balanced choices the rest of the week.

Important Message

The following food intake discussion can be a complement to nutritional recommendations from your doctor or dietitian. If you have any special digestive conditions, needs or any other stomach or intestinal conditions that restricts you from certain foods or behaviors then continue to follow the recommendations of your doctor or dietitian. Consult with your doctor or dietitian for clearance before any dietary changes. Dietitians are valuable professionals who can assist you with dietary recommendations specific to your needs especially if you are diabetic, overweight or have special medical conditions requiring specific dietary recommendations.

Not all foods or all food related issues have been discussed nor was it the purpose of this guide. The food suggestions and the purpose of the guide is to provide you with guidance regarding making balanced food choices in order to help you regain control of your diabetes and of your weight. For further details regarding food consumption consult with your doctor, dietitian, the American Diabetes Association and the American Dietetic Association.

Meal Structure Blueprint for All People Including Diabetics

How can you make food selections within the proportions of 50 to 55% carbs, 25-30% fats and 20-25% proteins in order to balance out these nutrients and lose weight permanently without dieting or deprivation? Here's how:

- Get familiar with this meal plan, food Lists A and B; go over them several times until you become very familiar with their content.
- This flexible meal plan is the cure to the "dieting" dilemma; it is based on having 3 main meals, 2 fruit snacks and 6-8 glasses of water per day. When you make food choices as suggested in "The Meal Plan," you will be consuming balanced proportions of foods from the 3 main nutrients: about 50-55% Carbs, 25-30% fat, and 20-25% protein (see List A for favorable sources from each food category). Aim at making about **5 choices daily from vegetables and fruits** (*make a different choice of fruit and vegetables each time in order to ensure that you are getting all the vitamins and nutrients necessary to prevent disease*), **and include two daily servings of dairy** (good sources of calcium and protein).
- **Chew slowly: It takes about 20 minutes** from the time you start chewing your meal for the brain to realize that you are getting full, so chew slowly and take your time eating. When you eat fast, within less than 20 minutes, you can gulp down massive amounts of food before your brain realizes you are full.
- *Portion sizes*: **For lunch and dinner food choices (as discussed in the "Meal Blueprint" below), limit portion sizes to an imaginary average round size dinner plate as follows:**

Whether eating in or out, picture an average round size plate and divide that round plate into 3 sections; one half section and 2 quarter sections:

1. Fill the half section with veggies (as a salad, cooked, or raw with veggie dip).
2. Fill one quarter section with lean meat (from the meat section in List A).
3. Fill the remaining quarter with high fiber/ complex Carbs (from the high fiber carbs section of List A).

No more weighing and no more guessing how much is enough no more guessing how many grams of this or that and no more counting calories. Attempting to count while consuming foods takes away the fun, spontaneity and pleasure of enjoying that food. This imaginary average round size plate distribution will give you a good gauge of balanced portion of foods to eat and at the same time it is filling. *More importantly this food distribution will give you an end to the guessing game of portion sizes.*

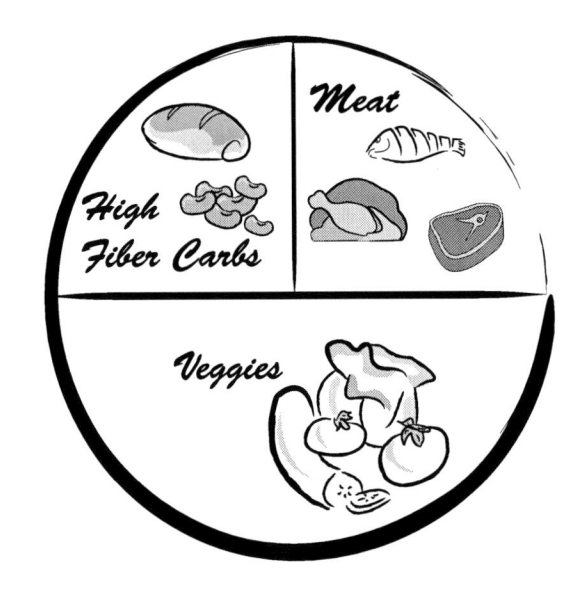

Portion Sizes (An Average Size Round Plate)

- While eating out, order wisely and stay within the limits of the food distribution of that imaginary average size round plate. Take the extra food home.

- While cooking your food, use lightly greased pans with good sources of liquid fat from List A; when choosing salad dressings, choose vinaigrettes which contain olive oil.

- **How much fat?** Even if "fat" is not mentioned in each of the meals, you will have balanced amounts of it nestled in the various food sources from which you will be choosing, such as: milk and cheeses, nuts, vinaigrette dressing (contains olive oil which help lower blood cholesterol when consumed in moderation about 2 to 3 teaspoonfuls on a salad) or other dressings; and fat is in the various meat and fish choices, as well as in avocados and various cooking oils, and is also found in many more food choices in the Fat choices in List A. Review the benefits of each of the food categories: Carbs, Fats, and Proteins discussed above.

- **Food items swap from List B to List A of your favorite recipes (keep all else same).** If some of your favorite recipes call for ingredients from List B (less favorable) then make the substitution to the same category of ingredients but from List A (more favorable). This "Meal Blueprint" structure, provided below, is not limiting, and it does not require you to stop eating the foods you grew up with. Rather, this meal structure gives you the flexibility of choosing and cooking the same food you are used to but with a healthier twist. Let's say your grandmother's favorite casserole recipe calls for 1 stick (a hypothetical amount) of butter to cook some of the other ingredients. Butter is an item in the Fats section of List B (food items in List B are less favorable for health if consumed daily) then make a healthier substitution from one the healthier Fats and Oils choices in List A. So in this case you decide to choose instead of butter, a tablespoonful of sunflower oil, which is a healthier choice. If that casserole recipe calls for white noodles or white pasta (found in List B Less Favorable Carbs) then make a substitution to one of the higher fiber carb options such as brown/ whole wheat pasta or noodles or barley (found in the high fiber/ complex Carbs section of List A). Keep all else about your grandmother's recipe the same. So on and so forth.

- **Always eat and choose food that tastes good**. Never sacrifice taste for any reason. Fat-free and sugar-free foods, snacks and dressings may not taste good; therefore, I would not recommend choosing them. When you choose a regular version of your favorite dressing or cheese and you eat it in smaller amounts, you will be a whole lot more satisfied and you won't have a sense of deprivation.

- You gain control of the foods you choose to eat when you keep your daily food distribution, content and portions (80% of the time) balanced. When you "get in the habit" of making healthy food choices (mostly from List A) whenever you eat out or cook in, and reduce your portion sizes (similar to the imaginary regular-sized round plate); You will enjoy the food you eat, you will ensure that you are consuming food from all the food groups in a balanced manner, you will get all the precious nutrients that help ward off disease, and you will lose weight without dieting. **That is a definition of a healthier more vibrant you.**

- **Apply what you learned in building a new habit** (in "What is a habit" discussion above) to making favorable food choices as outlined in the "Meal Blueprint" below. Remember, in the initial 3-4 weeks, you will forget, at times, to make "this" or "that" better food choice; but always remember the story about starting a new job and how uncomfortable you were initially; remember that you made mistakes but you corrected them and moved on. Also remember the example about your new car with new parking brake location; how initially you were still trying to reach out to the old location. After persistent trials and corrections you got it. Apply the same here. After 3-4 weeks, you will start making more favorable food choices and it becomes first nature to you; in other words, you will develop a new good habit of making good food choices most of the time. You will start losing weight and you will keep that weight off because this has become second-nature to you to make healthier food choices the majority of time. You have become in control of the food you eat. If occasionally (about 20% of time) you felt like controllably indulging then you do so without feeling guilty because the majority of time (about 80%) you were making good choices. This is non-restrictive, and you can go on doing this permanently.

- **Assess your results by weighing yourself once a week**. If you are not losing weight, ask yourself what food you are eating more frequently from List B in larger quantities? Then reverse the balance by making food choices less frequently and in smaller portions from List B and by making food selections the majority of time from all food categories from List A. Also, notice whether you have been skipping meals or snacks, then return to the " Meal Blueprint" structure below. **Account for all food and liquids that go in your mouth**: "Oh, I just had a "small" bag of cookies, or some chips (maybe a large bag), and I was thirsty so I drank a "small" bottle (16 ounces) of chocolate milk." Switch to snack choices from List A and switch to water. Moreover, if you are not losing weight, ask yourself whether you have become less active; then reverse the balance and do more walking during the day (refer to the activity section).

- **Don't be too harsh on yourself**, forgive yourself, love yourself and keep going. There is always the next day to make a better choice, but never, ever give up the relentless pursuit of what it takes to preserve your health.

- **Don't skip meals or snacks:** You can avoid being hungry and overeating at a meal when you don't skip any of the meals and snacks outlined in the "Meal Blueprint" structure below. When you have a solid base of 3 meals during the day, and you reinforce that base with a couple of fruit snacks in between as suggested below, then you are not only making sure that you are getting all the nutrients your body needs, but you also avoid going without food for more than 2-3 hours. So, when you get to the next meal or "buffet," you are not "get out of the way" hungry but are able to better control the kind of food and amounts of food you choose to make.

Remember, FEEL GUILT NO MORE since you are no longer dieting. You are a winner, any way you look at it, since you are freed from the cumbersome "diet" burden, and also freed of the limitation and guilt associated with counting calories or grams of this or that, or keeping track of which phase (1, 2 or 3) you are on of "Diet X or Z." You will enjoy the natural spontaneity of eating your meals "just like everyone else" without going overboard; you will still enjoy the same food/s you are used to with only minor changes that take place regarding portion size and food ingredient choices.

Dare to make that transition to a healthier, more fit you, and dare to age gracefully and enjoy an ultimate quality of life throughout this beautiful journey of life. It is as simple as ABC. So sit back and enjoy the ride of a lifetime.

The Meal Blueprint

BREAKFAST

Sample Choice #1

- Cereal of choice from List A (one serving as indicated on the cereal box) *and*
- Low fat milk or soy milk (enough to saturate the cereal) *and/or*
- 1 fruit (you may skip the fruit here and have it for a snack) *and*
- Coffee or tea (black or sweetened with Splenda) *and*
- 1 glass of water.

Sample Choice #2

- 1 slice of toasted whole grain bread (from List A) *and*
- Light cream cheese *and/or*
- 1 fruit *and*
- Coffee or tea (black or sweetened with Splenda) *and*
- 1 glass of water.

Sample Choice #3

- Once or twice a week.
- Two eggs (prepared your favorite way) or a veggie omelet (made with 2 eggs) *and*
- 1 slice of whole grain bread (from List A) (skip the butter or use very lightly) *and*
- 1 small pancake (you may add blueberry or walnuts, skip the butter or use very lightly) made with whole grain flour (if you want a couple pancakes then skip the bread) *and*
- Coffee or tea (black or sweetened with Splenda) *and*
- 1 glass of water.

Sample Choice #4

- Create your own meal with similar nutrient distribution and portions with choices of ingredients mostly from List A.

> **PS:**
> - Many restaurants offer whole grain bread, brown pasta and rice and pancakes made with whole grain flour, you just have to ask.
> - I deliberately did not include juices because they typically contain a high amount of sugar, and an 8-ounce glass may have the equivalent of 3 or 4 oranges or apples and is less filling. Eating whole fruit is more filling and has more fiber. If you must have juice with your breakfast, then a 4 to 6 ounces glass is fine.

SNACK

- 1 fruit from List A (make a different fruit choice every time) **and**
- 1 glass of ice water (lemon, lime, orange slice, or sugar free flavoring powders available in delicious multiple flavors, can be added to your water for flavor).

LUNCH

(See "Cooking methods" below for suggestions on cooking food other than frying)

Every meal needs to include a variety of veggies, a source of meat and a source of whole grain or a high fiber Carbs in the amounts of that imaginary average round size dinner plate; half a plate for the veggies, a quarter plate for lean meat or fish and the last quarter for the high fiber/complex carbs (for details on portion sizes refer to the 3rd point titled "Portion sizes" from the top of the previous section):

Veggies

- Grilled, boiled, raw, sautéed, stir fried, or as salad (from List A).
- Dressing: half to 1 packet of dressing, preferably a vinaigrette, Italian or French Ranch and Thousand Island are heavier. The thicker the dressing, the heavier the fat content. Start with a half packet then toss the salad to spread evenly. If more is needed then you can add a little more.
- Go easy on croutons (which are fried bread) or other breaded components, bacon and cheese.

Quantity/portion: Enough to cover a half section of that average round size dinner plate.

Proteins

- Choice of lean meat, pork, chicken or fish (from List A).
- Beans can be substituted if meat is not desired.

Quantity/portion: Select one choice of meat or a combination of two but enough to cover about a quarter section of that plate.

Whole Grains/High Fiber Carbs (from List A) such as:

- 1 or 2 slices of whole grain bread *or*
- Small baked potato with skin (go very easy (a smear) on the butter, sour cream, cheese or bacon) *or*
- Brown rice *or*
- Whole wheat pasta *or*
- Any other one choice of high fiber or grain products from the Carbs section of List A.

Quantity/portion: Choose one or multiple choices of high fiber carbs from List A, enough to cover the last quarter section of that average round size plate.

Beverages

- A glass of water *or*
- A diet soft drink *or*
- Iced tea (sweetened with Splenda or other sweeteners).

SNACK (FROM LIST A)

Sample Choice #1

- Mixed nuts (a half palm-ful) or (other choices of nuts from " Nuts and seeds" in the "Snacks" section towards the bottom of List A) *and*
- 1 fruit (different from fruits consumed earlier) *and*
- 1 glass of water.

Sample Choice #2

- Low-fat and low-sugar yogurt (small size 4 to 6 ounce cup) *and*
- Sprinkle in the yogurt a pinch or two of sunflower, pepitas, and soybean seed mix or almonds and nuts (these contain oils that can lower cholesterol and are heart friendly. See more choices in "Nuts and seeds" of "Snacks" towards the bottom of List A) *and*

- Two squares of dark chocolate *and*
- 1 glass of water.

Sample Choice #3

- One dairy choice (from list of "Favorable sources of dairy" below) *and*
- One slice whole grain bread or a couple crackers of whole grain "Triscuits" *and*
- 1 fruit (different from previous choices) *and*
- 1 glass of water.

> **PS: When a fruit (a form of sugar) is combined with balanced amounts of fat (couple pinches in the palm) of mixed nuts, seeds or dark chocolate, or a protein source, it makes the fruit go a longer way.** In the stomach and intestines, fat and/or protein makes the sugar break down at a slower rate consequently causing a mellower rise of sugar and lesser of a peak in your blood. **The net result: you won't get hungry as fast.**

DINNER
(See "Cooking methods" below for suggestions on cooking food other than by frying)

Make choices for dinner in the same structure and portions as for lunch; only choose a different variety of vegetables, meat, and high fiber carbs with every snack or meal to ensure you are getting a variety of all nutrients. Remember to limit portion sizes to that imaginary average round size dinner plate.

Veggies or Salad

- Same structure but different variety than lunch.

Quantity/portion: Enough to cover a half section of that average round size dinner plate.

Meat or Fish or Beans

- Same structure but different variety than lunch. Make choices 80 % of time from List A.

Quantity/portion: Select one choice of meat or a combination of two but enough to cover about a quarter section of that plate.

Whole Grain/High Fiber Carb

- Same structure but different variety than lunch from the Carbs section of List A. Make choices 80 % of time from List A.

Quantity/portion: Choose one or multiple choices of high fiber carbs from List A, enough to cover the last quarter section of that average round size plate.

Beverages

- A glass of water *or*
- Iced tea (sweetened with Splenda or other sweeteners).

Dessert

- 3 or 4 times a week
- Any small portion sizes of your favorable dessert choices in List A, such as a couple small scoops of no-added-sugar ice cream or desserts made with low sugar and fat. Occasionally, you can indulge with desserts from List B.

Water

- Don't forget to drink 6 to 8 glasses of water throughout each day.

Delicious Cooking Methods Other than Frying

There are several delectable ways to cook food besides frying. When cooking or ordering food out for any of the meals, choose (most days of the week) food that is:

- Grilled
- Steamed
- Boiled
- Baked
- Blackened (for fish mainly)
- Broiled
- Steamed
- Sautéed
- Stir fried (in small amounts of favorable oils listed in the "Fats" section of List A)
- Cooked with a pressure cooker
- Slowly cooked in a crock-pot

So as you see, frying is **not the only** and most delicious way to cook foods. Try these other healthier and more delicious ways to prepare food. Eat fried food less frequently (once or twice a week). Frying falls in List B, and all fried items should be consumed less frequently.

> **WHAT ABOUT SALT (TECHNICALLY KNOWN AS SODIUM)?**
>
> Go easy on salt when seasoning food or salad. Various components of the food you eat contain salt, so adding salt to your food may create an excess. Remember that excess salt raises blood pressure. Try not to exceed 3000 mg (read food labels of packaged snacks to find out how much salt that food contains.) If you have high blood pressure or heart disease your daily salt limit should be 2000 mg. Packaged food, snacks and TV dinners can have high amounts of salt or what is referred to as Sodium. Read the Nutrition Labels of the food you eat.

> ## List A
> ### *Favorable Food Choices from All Food Categories (Carbs, Fats, Proteins and Snacks) to Be Consumed As Discussed in the "The Meal Blueprint"*
>
> The lists of food provided in List A and B are not exhaustive. Other food choices are available in each category, which may not be listed here. These lists give you prolific listings of food choices and a sense of direction. If you are about to make a food choice not listed here, you will be more easily able to assess which category it belongs to from List A or List B, and consequently you will have a sense of how much to eat from it and how frequently. If it is a food from your ethnic background and belongs to any of the food categories in List A, then you know you can consume it more frequently throughout the week and vice versa to consume it less frequently per week if it belongs to List B. or if a recipe calls for several ingredients, some of which belong to List B, then you can choose to make substitutions to ingredients In List A of the same food category.

Carbs
Choices of Complex/High Fiber Carbs (Low in Sugar Content)

GREAT TASTING BREAKFAST CHOICES

Choose any one of these choices in the amount of one serving as indicated on the Nutrition Label of each product:

- FiberOne cereal (14 grams of fiber per serving and no sugar)
- Kashi brand cereal (several great tasting products; choose the ones containing less than 8 to 10 grams of sugar and anywhere from 5 to 13 grams of fiber)
- Quaker Oats bran
- Old fashioned oatmeal
- Kellogg's All-Bran with extra fiber
- Cooked oatmeal
- Kellogg's Bran Buds with Psyllium
- All Bran cereal
- Uncle Sam's with flaxseed brand cereal
- Whole wheat pancake mix (Aunt Jemima and Kodiak cakes by Baker Mills, 100% whole grain flour used)
- Raisin Bran
- Bran Buds
- Oats
- Cereal containing barley, buckwheat and/or rye
- Any breakfast or cereal bar that is low in total calories (about 150 calories), low in total carbs (about 18 to 20 gm), low in sugar (about 7 or 8 gm), high fiber (7 to 10 or more), low in sugar alcohols (2-4 gm), balance in fat (4-5 gm), balance in protein (5-7 gm)

> **PS:** You can mix smaller quantities to equal about 1 serving from 2 or more cereal products if some have more fiber and less sugar than others in order to improve taste.

BREAD CHOICES

- Whole grain bread
- Whole grain pumpernickel
- Whole wheat pita
- Sourdough rye
- Rye
- Mutli-Grain flour Tortillas (by Mission; **4 grams fiber** per Fajita size tortilla)
- Whole grain (or wheat) bagel
- Whole grain (or wheat) muffin
- Sourdough

RICE, PASTA, BEAN PRODUCTS, AND OTHER GRAIN CHOICES

- Brown rice
- Long grain wild rice
- Basmati rice
- Dirty rice
- Rice Pilaf
- Barley
- Baked potato with skin (little butter and sour cream used) (medium size is portion)
- Sweet potatoes with skin
- Brown whole wheat pasta (all pasta, spaghetti and noodle versions)

BEAN PRODUCTS

- Green beans
- Kidney beans
- Pinto beans
- Pole beans
- Red beans
- Black beans
- Black-eyed peas
- Beans
- Garbanzo or chick peas
- Lima beans
- Soy beans
- Peas
- Lentils
- All other beans not listed here

OTHER GRAIN PRODUCTS WITH HIGH FIBER CONTENT

- Couscous
- Stone ground corn meal
- Cracked wheat (bulgur)
- Buckwheat
- Sweet corn

Fats and Oils

CHOICES OF FOODS CONTAINING HIGHLY HEALTHY AND FAVORABLE FATS

These include unsaturated fats and fats which contain Omega-3 and Omega-6, which are known for their heart-protective properties; they reduce cholesterol and thin the blood. They must be consumed 4-5 times weekly (at least) but in small amounts (to avoid weight gain).

OMEGA-3 OR OMEGA-6 CONTAINING OILS

These can withstand heat and are mostly used for cooking. **Use about 2 to 3 teaspoonfuls or so** of any oil to cook foods on stovetop or in the oven:

- Flaxseed oil
- Cod-liver oil
- Walnut oil
- Sesame oil
- Soybean oil
- Corn oil
- Cottonseed oil
- Sunflower oil
- Safflower oil

OTHER FAVORABLE OILS WHICH LOWER CHOLESTEROL

Mostly used in salads and for sautéing purposes over medium to light heat equivalent to the amount about 2 to 3 teaspoonfuls drizzled over a salad or used in a pan for sautéing purposes:

- Canola oil (can withstand heat and can be used for cooking)
- Avocado oil
- Grape seed oil
- Olive oil

OTHER FAVORABLE SOURCES OF FATS AND OILS:

- Olives
- Tahini (sesame paste)
- Avocados
- Tofu
- Peanut butter (one tablespoon)

Protein

LEAN SOURCES OF MEATS (POULTRY, PORK, AND BEEF)

- Chicken
- Cornish hen
- Duck
- Quail
- Pheasant
- Goose
- Rabbit
- Venison
- Buffalo
- Ground beef with less than 10-20% fat
- Flank steak
- T-bone
- Roast, chuck and round steaks
- Porterhouse
- Lean cuts of meat (all meats with names that end in "oin" such as tenderloins and sirloins)
- Ground round
- Canadian bacon
- Pork tender
- Pork center loin chop
- Pork top loin
- Pork chop
- Pork cutlet
- Roast pork butt
- Veal chop
- Veal roast
- Veal cutlet
- Lamb roasts
- Lamb chop
- Leg of lamb
- Lamb rib roast
- Ground lamb
- Lean cuts of deli (low fat ham, chicken turkey and lean meat)

FISH PRODUCTS (CONTAINING OMEGA-3)

Consume 4 to 5 times a week:

- Salmon
- Mackerel
- Sardines
- Clams
- Crab
- Lobster
- Scallops
- Shrimp
- Tuna
- Halibut
- Cod
- Flounder
- Haddock
- Herring
- Catfish
- Oysters

Veggies

Consume these veggies up to 3 to 5 times or more if possible. Eat them raw with or without vegetable dips, as snacks (tomatoes, cucumbers, broccoli, cauliflower, green peppers), lightly steamed, cooked in stews, baked along with roasts or sautéed with a drizzle of olive oil; veggies must remain hard in texture to retain nutrients. When overcooked, they can lose many nutritive values.

- Broccoli
- Lettuce (all types)
- Tomatoes
- Brussels sprouts
- Cucumbers
- Peppers (all colors and types)
- Onions
- Garlic
- Carrots
- Celery
- Celery roots
- Spinach
- Beets
- Collards
- Turnip greens
- Kale
- Swiss chard
- Sweet potatoes
- Cauliflower
- Squash
- Okra
- Eggplant
- Asparagus
- Palmitto
- Greens
- All other vegetables not listed here

The benefits of vegetables are endless and cannot be replaced with a supplement pill. Numerous studies have shown that vegetables have loads of nutrients, vitamins and fiber, and assist in heart-protective functions, and contribute to weight loss. Some, such as okra and eggplants also contain plant sterols and "Flavonoids" that can help the body rid itself of some bad cholesterol thus reducing its concentration in the blood and around the arteries. A most recent study published in *The American Journal of Clinical Nutrition* in June 2005, showed (after a follow-up study of 55,000 Swedish women) that when these women consumed plant foods and whole grain foods and ate less animal products, they had drastically fewer incidents of obesity and showed that they controlled their weight on a long-term basis.

Favorable Choices of Dairy Products

Consume twice daily any of the choices below. Each serving size for solid cheese is the equivalent of 3 stackable fingers, half to 1 cup for milk, and 4 to 6 ounces for yogurt, 2 teaspoonfuls for cream cheese.

Dairy products are essential sources of Calcium and protein. Regular cheese with the exception of Cottage, Ricotta and the "Light" version of cheeses contain up to 80% or more saturated (bad fats). This is why it is best to consume the more favorable dairy sources such as low fat milk, low fat and low sugar yogurt, and the light (low fat or part-skim) version of the other cheese twice daily in the amounts suggested above.

No one can deny the delectable qualities of cheeses produced here at home or French or other European cheeses. How about eating those in balanced amounts 20% of time or once or twice a week? Does that sound fair?

- Milk (skim, 1 or 2%)
- All cheeses (the light version or part-skim version preferred 80% of time)
- Cream cheese (light)
- Light yogurt (with unsweetened fruit chunks or sweetened with sugar substitute)

Snacks, Desserts & Beverages

Fruit Choices

Non-ripe fruit; eat it hard, as the sugar content increases after they become ripe. Eating whole fruits is preferred over canned fruits and fruit juices, due to their high sugar content.

Eat fruits 2 to 3 times daily as outlined in "The Meal Blueprint" above. One medium size fruit is the average portion size for bulky fruits such as bananas, oranges, pears and apples. For smaller size fruits such as apricots and prunes, 2 to 3 constitute a portion size. For small size fruits such as grapes or any fruit from the berry family, then a half-cup is a balanced portion size. For melons and tropical fruits cut in cubes, half to one cup is an appropriate portion size.

- Apples with skin
- Bananas
- Oranges and all other citrus fruits
- Peaches with skin
- Apricots
- Grapes
- Pears with skin
- Watermelon
- Cantaloupes (and all the melon family)
- Grapefruit
- Strawberries
- Blackberries and all the berry family
- Blueberries (have the highest antioxidant content of any fruit)
- Avocado (contain heart friendly fat but are high in fat amounts. Eat in moderation one medium size up 2 to 4 times a week).
- Prunes
- Cherries
- Kiwi
- Mango
- Pineapple
- Papaya
- All tropical fruits except coconuts and dates (eat those less frequently since they contain saturated fats)
- Plums
- Dried fruit (unsweetened) (figs, raisins, apricots, dates and others) in small quantities (a portion size is 2 to 4 pieces depending on fruit size)
- All other fruits not mentioned here

Nuts and Seeds

Some containing Omega-3 and other Fats that Lower Cholesterol and all a great source of Vitamin E. Portion size: About half a palm-full a day. Select choices of nuts unsweetened and not containing honey:

- Almonds (Omega-3)
- Walnuts (Omega-3)
- Cashews
- Mixed nuts
- Sunflower seeds
- Pumpkin seeds
- Pecans
- Peanuts
- Macadamia
- Flaxseed (Omega-3)
- Sesame
- Wheat germ
- Soybeans

Favorable Desserts and Snacks that Are Low In Sugar and High in Fiber:

- Raisin oat bran muffins
- Oat bran muffins and walnuts
- Oat bran muffins
- Packaged snacks that are high in fiber and low in sugar such as: **Triscuits** baked whole grain crackers and a portion (the size of 3 stacked fingers) of your favorite cheese
- Pancakes made with whole grain wheat, flour and whole grain oat flour along with walnuts (contain Omega-3 heart oil source) and blueberries (contain the highest concentrations of heart protective antioxidant vitamins. Use sugar free syrup or small drizzles of maple syrup.)
- Apple muffins
- Pound cake
- Cakes made with Splenda or made with low sugar content or sweetened with fruits

Favorable Dessert Choices:

- Ice cream with no sugar added and low in fat (read and compare labels)
- Low-carb and low-calorie cookies and chocolate bars with "Net Carb" content ranging from 0-5 grams. Some brands are Carborite and Ross
- Dark chocolate (2 to 3 small squares per day)
- Angel cakes (small wedge)
- Pudding made with little or no sugar or sweetened with natural sugar, Splenda, or sugar alcohols (small cup)
- Small portion of any cake or a small muffin made with low sugar, fruit or dried raisins and containing **no "Trans Fat."** Nuts, dark chocolate chips, whole grain flour or oat bran can be used.

> **DRINKS CONTAINING NO SUGAR:**
>
> - Water (carbonated or regular, with or without sugar free powdered flavors)
> - Flavored water with no sugar
> - Tea or iced tea (using sweetener) (limit yourself to a couple daily)
> - Coffee (using sweetener) (limit yourself to a couple daily)
> - Diet soft drink (limit yourself to a couple drinks daily)

> ## List B
>
> These are less favorable choices of all food groups, namely Carbs, fats, proteins and snacks and to be consumed once or twice a week as discussed in "The Meal Blueprint." Foods in List B, if consumed regularly and more frequently per week will contribute to weight gain and to raising the risk of artery and heart disease, and consequently raising the incidence of heart attacks and strokes.
>
> ### CARBS
>
> Carbs in this List B are high in sugar and low in fiber. These food choices are less favorable for your health since they are stripped of most nutrients, vitamins and fiber and contribute to weight gain and disease if consumed many days of the week. They are high in sugar; they have very low nutritive value, and are loaded with calories. However, if you

eliminate them from your diet you will crave them more. Making food choices from this group once or twice a week in balanced portion sizes (similar to their List A counterparts, may be part of a balanced lifestyle).

- All cereal with sugar content over 8 to 10 grams and fiber content less than 3 grams per serving as per box label
- White rice
- Instant rice
- Breaded ingredients for batter
- White bread (all white bread products including biscuits and corn bread)
- White pasta (all white pasta and noodles)
- Popcorn
- Corn bread
- Rice cake
- French fries
- Wonder Bread
- Croutons and other breaded components that could be sprinkled over a salad
- Bagels
- Baked potatoes (without skin and includes loads of butter, sour cream, cheese and bacon all of which are saturated fats and contribute to clogging your arteries)
- Mashed potatoes
- Pizzas
- English muffins
- All other processed foods containing refined sugar products not mentioned here
- White tortillas

Your tastes have adapted to the high sugar content in these foods. If you make the switch to the list of breads and carbs in List A, in a matter of a few days, your taste will adapt to the low sugar content and the healthier food selection from List A. You will wonder how you liked those foods with a high sugary taste in them.

FATS AND OILS

List B choices of fats and oils is least favorable for health and contribute to the formation of Plaques around the artery walls restricting, gradually, the flow of blood to your precious organs; your heart and brain. Consequently, these fats and oils in List B promote heart disease, worsening of current disease conditions and promote weight gain if consumed on regular basis more than once or twice a week.

Portion sizes of about a teaspoonful of butter, or margarine, or sour cream can be smeared over your baked potato should you so desire once or twice a week. The same applies to mayonnaise where a teaspoonful or two can be used to smear with burgers or sandwiches once or twice a week. The rest of the time mustard, ketchup or both can be used the majority of time. Occasionally you can go slightly more. About two teaspoonfuls is the limit to cook with these fats once or twice a week. The rest of times use fats and oils from List A.

- Solid fats (all solid fats such as butter or margarine)
- Trans fats (found in some packaged foods. Please read Nutrition Labels)
- Lard or any other pork fat
- Shortenings
- Palm oil
- Coconut oil
- Mayonnaise (the light version is preferred)
- Sour cream
- Any other animal fat or processed solid fat not listed here

Proteins

Unfavorable choices of meats and protein containing high amounts of saturated fats and cholesterol and can contribute to heart and artery disease and weight gain just like it is discussed in the previous "Fats and Oils" discussion portion and need to be limited to once or twice a week in portions as outlined in "The Meal Blueprint." Having said that, who is going to pass a delicious Filet Mignon or a delicious cut of steak at a nice steakhouse occasionally? Not me. Moderation and balance is key to food enjoyment.

- All "Western meals" (cheeseburgers, fries, soft drinks, hot dogs, pizza etc..) unless modified as discussed in "Western Meal Makeover" below)
- All fried foods
- Bacon and bacon bits found in salad bars
- All Fatty cuts of steaks and meats such Filet Mignon, New York strip and many other marbled meat cuts
- Fatty cuts of pork
- Organ meats
- Fatty hams
- Ground beef containing more than 10% fat
- Spare ribs pork
- Sausage patties and links
- Pepperoni
- Fatty cuts of deli such as Mortadella, Bologna, Salami, Prosciutto
- Hot dogs (except the Healthy Choice brands or any brand that is low in saturated fats and total fat content)
- Beef sausage (except Healthy Choice brands or any other brand that contains low saturated fats and low total fat content)
- Egg yolks (no more than 4 or 5 egg yolks per week. You may consume more egg white as it is 100% pure protein with no fat or cholesterol)
- Beef ribs

DAIRY PRODUCTS

These have high amounts of saturated fats and need to be consumed no more than once or twice weekly, should you desire so.

- Heavy cream
- Whole milk
- Heavy milk byproducts
- Buttermilk
- Cheeses (all non reduced version of solid and cream cheeses)

DESSERT AND SNACKS

Consume infrequently once or twice per week or make selections form List A desserts and consume more frequently:

- Ice cream
- Processed and packaged cookies
- Peanut butter
- Processed and packaged pastries
- Processed and packaged cakes
- Snack crackers, chips and all packaged snacks
- All candy and confectionary products
- All packaged cookies, "breakfast bars" and desserts that have a sugar content of more than 8 to 10 grams and less than 3 grams of fiber per serving as per the Nutrition Label
- All heavy creams (unless available in low fat versions)
- Non-dairy whipped cream (unless available in low fat versions)
- Granola bars
- Sweetened chocolate and milk chocolate containing bars
- All cakes, icing, candy bars, cookies, and pies
- Cheesecakes
- Table sugar
- Honey
- Jams
- Cakes, cookies and pies
- Croissants
- Pancakes (made with white flour)
- Pancake, maple or sugar syrup
- Vanilla wafers
- Doughnuts
- All other desserts and sweets not mentioned here

DRINKS (LESS FAVORABLE FOR HEALTH):

- All soft drinks (the biggest contributor (up to 33%) to obesity in the USA).
- All fruit juices and orange juice when consumed most days of the week. Fruit juices contain added sugar. Eating whole fruit is a better option than drinking fruit juice. One 8 ounce glass of orange or apple juice is the equivalent of 3 to 4 pieces of fruit that are squeezed and stripped of the fiber you get when you eat the whole fruit. May consume about 6 ounces 2 or 3 days a week should you so desire. Cut back one fruit consumption that day.

Lifestyle Choices

> - Fruit punch.
> - All "Energy" drinks (they contain loads of sugar and caffeine and have the potential to **dangerously** raise blood pressure in people with blood pressure and heart problems and can cause major strokes and heart attacks when combined with prescription drugs such as antidepressants, some drugs for migraine, appetite suppressants and Over The Counter decongestants and some herbals).

General Food Selection Tips:

- Be creative. Nothing is cast in stone. You may select breakfast choices, which include high-fiber cereals as snacks.

- Remember to aim at balance and avoid perfection. When you make a not-so- favorable choice or two, forgive yourself and make a better choice the next day; remain persistent in improving your "lifestyle choices." It's easy.

- Make food selections, most of the time, (about 80% of the time) from List A.

- Do not deprive yourself from foods and snacks in List B, but make choices from each of its categories "less frequently," about 20% of the time or once or twice a week.

- Make a variety of food choices each time you choose foods. In other words, if for lunch you chose a salad containing lettuce, tomato and cucumbers, then for your vegetable choice for dinner, you can select raw vegetables such as broccoli, celery, and carrots along with a vegetable dip. or you can choose to have stir-fried vegetables at a Chinese restaurant. If, for your mid-day snack, you chose an apple as your fruit choice, then for the mid-afternoon snack, you might select a banana, strawberries or an orange for your fruit choice.

- Always cook or select foods that taste good. Never sacrifice taste. However, your taste will adapt to a diet soft drink and to foods that are low in sugar and fat after your repeated exposure to them. Later on, when you do taste highly sweetened foods and foods high in fat, such as you'd eaten before, you will wonder how you were able to eat such heavy foods. Great tasting food is not always made with heavy fats but incorporate a delicate balance of every ingredient.

- Remember to reduce portion sizes regardless of any food you are consuming. Remember any excess amount of food can turn into fat, even if it is from List A. Any favorable source of food, consumed in large amounts and consumed frequently, can turn into "junk food."

- **To avoid overeating at dinner parties, buffets, or at holiday feasts, have a snack from the "Snacks" choices in List A approximately 1½ hours to 2 hours prior to that meal. This way, you prevent overeating, and you can make more balanced selections when in presence of that feast.**
- **You can add to the foods in List A; add foods from your own ethnic or cultural backgrounds, provided they are favorable sources of whole grain, and provided they are high in fiber, low in sugar, and rich in heart-protecting fats and low in heart-damaging and disease-contributing fat.**

People gain weight by excessively eating foods that belong to the same food groups during each meal or snack and stray away from limiting portions most of the time. For instance, say you are eating out at an American Buffet-style restaurant (**See how you can make better food choices and substitutions when eating out in a variety of restaurants in the section entitled "Meal Makeovers On The Go" next**). When you fill your 3 plates with loads of fried and breaded chicken, fried and breaded fish, a couple of pieces of fried and breaded chicken steaks, fried and breaded okra, French fries, two pieces of corn bread, one biscuit drenched with butter, three different kinds of desserts and ice cream, and you carry this wobbling "Tower of Pisa" to your seat, and you get a large iced tea and you sweeten that with 3 packets of sugar...

ASK YOURSELF THE FOLLOWING QUESTIONS:
- **Is this balance?**
- **Are these food choices I made mostly from List B or List A?**
- **And how do the portion sizes fit with that regular-size round plate where you fill half with vegetables, a quarter with lean meat, chicken, pork or fish and the remaining quarter with high fiber Carbs such as whole grain bread or beans or brown rice or brown pasta?**
- **Did I overdo it with the Carb group when I duplicated several choices from the same group, such as fried and breaded everything?**
- **Was there anything high-fiber in any of these choices which belong to List A?**
- **Will I likely gain weight and have all the health problems we have been talking about when I make food choices in this manner?**

One thing you must realize is, if you have a "craving" for a certain type of food, such as fried food or dessert, then have a small portion of it! It will satisfy your brain "and" your stomach, you do not need to overdo it. For instance, do you think it would have been a better choice to have started with a small salad with your favorite raw vegetables from the bar and your favorite dressing (go easy on the quantity) enough to fill a half-plate, then perhaps a couple of small strips of fried chicken and a couple of small strips of fish, enough to fill an imaginary quarter-plate; then for the remaining quarter, how about some pinto beans or green beans and "a few" fries; and if you "have to have" your cornbread, then how about only one small piece? You can have a biscuit next time. If you feel like having something sweet, you can top it all off with a small piece of rich brownie and skip everything else. For your drink, how about lemon in your tall ice water or a large iced tea sweetened with "Splenda" (which provides you with the same taste of sugar but without the calories, and minus the aftertaste other sweeteners might have). With these choices, you would have satisfied your cravings and will have made balanced food choices from all the food groups, in balanced proportions.

How to Assess the Portion Sizes of Food Recipes Which Contain a Number of Food Groups (Stews, Casseroles, Dinner Soups, Lasagna, Etc.)

Keep in mind that imaginary average round size dinner plate where veggies fill half, meats fill a quarter and high fiber carbs fill the remaining quarter.

EXAMPLE # 1: MEAT STEW WITH BARLEY AND BEANS

If you are eating meals that contain a combination of food categories, then find out which food group is missing from that round plate, and add it to your meal. For instance, say you are consuming a stew that contains beans, meats, and barley (if that stew originally called for white noodles {Carb from List B} then substitute with Barley {high fiber Carb from List A). That meal contains meat, which represents the meat group, barley, and beans represent the Carb group, what would then be missing from that meal is vegetables? So you can eat about one half a plate's worth of stew since a quarter plate will have the fiber from the beans and the barley, and the other quarter contains the mixed-in-meat. Then for the rest of the half plate, you can add a salad (take out the croutons because they are fried bread, and the Carb group is already in your meal in the form of barley and beans) and top that salad with your favorite dressing (go easy on the dressing or choose a vinaigrette, French or Italian). If you have not had a second portion of cheese that day, then you can sprinkle a little of your favorite cheese on top of the salad.

Example # 2: Meat Lasagna

Say you are in the mood for meat lasagna. Preferably, you should prepare or order the brown or whole-wheat form of that lasagna or pasta dish; whole wheat has much more fiber than its white cousin and it is in List A. Lasagna contains some dairy as it uses cheeses; it contains some fat from the meat and cheese; it contains the high-fiber Carbs from the brown pasta; and it contains meat. The only missing foods from that imaginary average round size plate are the vegetables. So you can have a square of lasagna to cover about half of the round plate (a quarter for the meat and a quarter for the Carbs but because they are mixed together they make a half) and then you can also add vegetables sautéed in a drizzle (small amount about 2 teaspoonfuls) of olive oil (great choice of fat that lowers cholesterol and protects the heart in the process) or in a raw form of your favorite vegetables with a little veggie dip, or in a salad form with a vinaigrette dressing.

Example # 3: Vegetable and Meat Soup

If you are consuming soup for a meal and if that soup contains potatoes, vegetables, beans and either chicken or meat, then you can consume a soup bowl, which will contain foods from all food groups.

Meal Makeovers When Eating Out

You are not alone if, when eating out, your usual order consists of a comforter-sized breaded chicken fried steak swimming in a pool of gravy or a 4-piece fried breaded chicken meal that lies next to a mountain of mashed potatoes, the tip of which is dented with a pool of heavy gravy along with a side of French fries and a buttered roll, all of which are served in an oblong-shaped mega-sized plate. The next time you eat out, instead of feeling the obligation of devouring these enormous feasts in one sitting, here are some tips that will help you make more balanced choices while eating out at restaurants.

How to Modify Meals When Eating Out and Make Them More Balanced

Burger Combo Makeover

It's a typical workday, and it is lunchtime. Although it is best not to select fast food restaurants on a daily basis, once or twice a week may be okay, as well as convenient. You are now inside the fast food joint and about to make your meal choice. You are faced with several meal combo choices of burgers and chicken. There's also a menu for salads, side orders and individual burgers not included in the combo meal choices. You are in the mood for a burger and fries combo. Here's how you do the makeover:

- Skip the double and triple-decker and bacon burger choices.
- Limit fries to once or twice a week.
- Select a hamburger combo with a diet soda as your drink.
- Skip the mayo and butter on the bread (there's enough fat from the meat and fries)
- Substitute mayo with mustard.
- Occasionally skip the cheese (when you feel like having cheese, then eat fewer fries).
- Keep all the veggies and condiments that come with it.
- Do not super-size any meal (remember that you are practicing smaller portion sizes).
- The order is not complete yet. What is still missing? The vegetables. Always have vegetables or salad with every meal. So, you order a green salad with your favorite dressing (you can choose a light dressing only if it tastes good.) Otherwise, you use the regular dressing of your choice and try not to use the whole pack or you can use a vinaigrette, Italian or French, a better and tasty choice. A tiny amount of dressing, once it's tossed, will cover the whole salad. Skip the croutons, since you will have some bread and fries (and there will be plenty of fat so you don't need additional fried bread). If you are dying for croutons, then have some and eat fewer fries.

Now it is time to eat. Before you do so, you can customize the meal even further:

- Trim the edges of both pieces of the burger bread (since you will have enough Carbs from the fries).
- Use half or three quarters of the packet of that Ranch or Thousand Island dressing and toss the salad. The dressing will be all over the salad, and you will have saved some unwanted additional calories.
- Start with the salad, so you can fill up on the vegetables first. Then finish off the rest of the meal and enjoy your food.

Grilled Chicken Combo Makeover

Next time you go to the fast food joint, instead of selecting a burger combo, how about a grilled chicken sandwich, a salad with beans tossed in it (if available), and a diet soft drink or ice water? Follow the same suggestions as above on everything; only this time, instead of the fries:

- Substitute with onion rings or chili.

Higher-End Burger Joint with Open Condiment Bars (Such as Fuddruckers):

- Fish is on the menu, and it is prepared in a couple of different ways: blackened, Cajun-style, and grilled. Burgers and chicken sandwiches are also on the menu. However, since fish is on the menu, you decide to order it Cajun-style, along with a small onion ring.
- Skip the fried fish.
- Skip the white bread and ask for whole grain bread (if available).
- Instead of ordering a salad, load up on the vegetables in the open bar, such as: lettuce, tomato, onions, pickles, jalapenos, mustard, catsup, and other healthy condiments.
- Add beans or chickpeas to the salad or to your veggie collection if they're available in order to raise the amount of fiber and other precious nutrients to your meal.

Hoagie or Deli Style Restaurants Meal Makeover (Such as a Subway or Quiznos)

You can select from various types of breads. Select whole grain, whole wheat, sourdough or rye bread, whichever is available and skip the butter on the bread and Mayonnaise on the bread. Order a one-foot-long sandwich (go ahead, with a one-foot choice of bread; it will undergo a makeover). Select the meat of your choice, go easy on the cheese, and request all the vegetables available to go on the sandwich along with some seasoning. Skip or go easy on the dressing options or oils that could be added to that sandwich. If you don't have the option of having the vegetables on the sandwich then order a side salad with Vinaigrette dressing and start the meal eating that salad. Skip the chips because you will be eating part of the whole grain from that sandwich. Chips (fried potatoes less the skin) belong to the carb family like the whole grain bread and will be an excess that may contribute to weight gain.

When it's time to eat, dissect the sandwich in the following manner. You can open the hoagie up and then eat the content (with a fork), including the meats and all the veggies in it. Of the whole foot-long whole-grain bread, you can eat a quarter or so of it and dump the rest. What you had done here is that you have taken advantage of all the additional veggies that came on that foot long without consuming excessively the entire bread. For a variation next time, you can order a 6-inch sandwich with the meat of your choice and give it the same makeover you did for the foot-long regarding the added veggies and eat the whole thing. If you like having a small bag of chips then go ahead but take out a part of that bread. For a drink a good choice would be a diet soft drink or ice water.

Pizza Makeover

When ordering a pizza, order thin-crust dough. Try to avoid ordering all the meats that are available, such as pepperoni, sausage and others. They are loaded with saturated fatty acids that are bad for your heart. You can order all the vegetables you'd like: onions, green peppers, olives, mushrooms and jalapenos. For the choice of meat, you can order Canadian bacon, since it is a leaner form of ham; order Canadian bacon on half the pizza and beef on the other. Ask the pizza operator to go easy on the cheese. When it's time to eat consume about 2-3 pieces. Limit the consumption of pizza to about once or twice per week. Pizza is listed in List B of food choices. Most importantly, you do not want to compromise the taste of that pizza; and if you do as suggested, the taste will not be compromised. Guaranteed.

Italian Meal Makeover

Whenever you order Italian, you expect pasta to be included in just about every order that is available. So the first thing you do is ask the waiter to substitute the white pasta with whole grain pasta or brown pasta. Then you can select any choice of meat, chicken or shrimp prepared in your favorite recipe. You can also choose veal, beef, eggplant Parmesan, or spaghetti and meatballs, lasagna or any other favorite choice. Don't forget the veggies or the salad. Always order a green salad and request for it to be served first. Always, when eating out, remember that all food groups need to be consumed in balance. Remember the average round size dinner plate, half of that plate is filled with veggies or a salad, a quarter is the meat choice, and the other quarter is the whole grain or high-fiber Carb choice.

When the food is served, you start eating the salad first to fill up on it. When you get the pasta, usually restaurants serve large portions of pasta, meats, chicken and everything else. Remember the portion sizes on a dinner plate and that you're practicing reducing portion sizes. A quarter of a dinner plate would be the whole grain pasta. Whatever remains, take it home in a box with you. The same applies to the meat portion. Eat about a quarter-size plate of that meat or chicken, and take the rest home. You can end that meal with a small dessert of your choice. If the dessert is oversized, then you can share it with your companion or take the rest home.

American Style Buffet Makeover

Important message: Prior to open buffet type meals if you eat a small snack (any from List A such as some mixed nuts and a fruit) about 45 minutes to an hour before that buffet you will control better your food choices and portion sizes and consequently eat a more balanced meal.

In a typical buffet, you're going to have about 20-30 items: all types of meats, vegetables, pizzas, you name it it's there. But how do you limit yourself to balanced portion sizes? Once at that buffet- style restaurant, remember the average round size dinner plate. Half of the plate is filled with veggies and salads, a quarter of the plate is filled with your meat portion, and the remaining quarter is filled with high fiber Carbs, such as whole grain bread, brown rice, beans or any other foods in List A. Try to make less fried and breaded choices of chicken or fish because of the bread component (you will be over-consuming your bread and Carb groups over the quarter size plate if you don't watch out for that).

However, if you occasionally wish to have a bigger serving of fried chicken, then reduce the portion of the Carb group. The same applies to your choice of bread; if you wish to combine mashed potatoes and a biscuit, just reduce the portion of the potatoes. They should fit approximately a quarter of your dinner plate. Keep in mind that the bean products contain the complex carbohydrates that fulfill the quarter portion of your dinner plate of Carbs. When it comes to the dessert section, if you feel like trying the various desserts that they have, then you can eat a bite or two of a couple of your favorite desserts, and it will be enough to satisfy your sweet tooth. Don't forget the water or iced tea sweetened with a sweetener.

Mexican Meal Makeover

If you feel like having Mexican food, then choices like fajitas, or Carne Guisada and Carnitas make the best choices since they have a balance of all ingredients. Mixed fajitas (chicken and beef) with beans (ask for the beans or frijoles; a better choice than refried beans), rice and avocados make a good combination. Limit yourself to 1-2 tortillas with that meal. Limit chips and salsa to just a few. If you consume a few chips and salsa at the beginning of the meal, then limit yourself to 1 tortilla with the fajita meal. When selecting other choices such as burritos, Chimichangas, any kind of rolled tortilla or taco-style food, remember to limit your consumption of the bread products to about 1 or 2. Remember the average round dinner plate, filling half of the plate with any veggies that are available, and then a quarter plate filled up with a meat product, and then the rest in whole grains, such as beans/frijoles.

Chinese Buffet Makeover

A typical Chinese buffet will have anywhere from 20-40 items in the buffet. Remember the dinner plate principle anywhere you go. Now you're going to have a lot of fried elements in that buffet. It's going to be hard to skip those fried egg rolls or the different types of breaded and fried products included there. You can consume some fried foods that you like in smaller portion sizes, but you're going to have to skip the rice when choosing, chicken, beef, pork or fish prepared in various styles with vegetables, often above rice. Just skip the rice. Start by having egg drop soup or sweet and sour soup, and then consume the small fried foods item you put on your plate. After you consume what you have on your plate, make another round to the buffet.

You're going to be making selections from the meat, seafood or chicken choices that are available, to fill about a half or three quarters of your plate, because vegetables are included in these preparations and you need to account for the vegetable portion here. In terms of whole grain, there may not be much whole grain products in a Chinese buffet but almost always you will find green beans and veggies that are cooked in the meal, such as the broccoli, celery, and others, are also rich in fiber. When it comes to the dessert, as in the American buffet counterpart, select 1-2 bites of a couple of desserts to satisfy your craving.

Free Joker Evening

You have made favorable choices all week long, and you are so proud of yourself for sticking with it week after week. So it's Friday night, and you're meeting up with some friends, and you select any restaurant of your choice. And I would try to have a controlled type of indulgence. If you are craving a certain kind of food, then now is the time to order it. Don't hold back, but stay within a controlled type of indulgence; this is not a time to go on a binge, and you will not have a need to do so since you have not been deprived of anything. Stay within the general guidelines of a vegetable component, a meat component, and a whole grain component. And if there's no whole grain, it's okay if you have white bread, or French baguette and butter as a starter, along with an appetizer of your choice. It's okay if you go overboard slightly with portion sizes. At the end, if you feel like having that decadent dessert with chocolate fudge or any other dessert you desire, go ahead and order it. But try to watch the portion size. Remember, you have been practicing portion control, and maybe now is also the time to do it, even if you go slightly overboard. If you got an oversized piece of dessert, share it with your companion.

Keeping a Daily Food Log

Keeping a daily food log, initially, 3-4 days a week, for only the first 2-3 weeks, is a great idea. It helps you track the food, and makes you aware of the kinds of food and portions sizes you are eating. Start recording your current daily food patterns for a day or two before you start recording your improved lifestyle choices as we discussed in this entire food section. Then start recording improved choices and portion sizes of foods and snacks you eat. If you make a not-so- favorable choice, then write down, next to it, a better choice you could have made, and make it next time. See a sample Food Log at the end of the guide. **You can make copies of the blank Food Log page for daily food tracking.**

ACTIVITY

Making Balanced Activity Choices
(Before starting any activity consult with your doctor first for clearance)

People have become more accustomed to sitting and inactivity all day long. From the desk jobs, to surfing the internet, to shopping online nowadays, to playing video games, to using elevators, to reading, to watching TV and movies on DVDs, people more than ever have become more and more sedentary. Beware; inactivity is a major magnet for disease as we age. People on a daily basis sit…sit….sit and conserve…conserve…conserve energy. The net result is obesity and disease. Instead, the opposite should be happening for improving health and warding off disease. So move…move… move and expand… expand….expand. The net result; regain control of your weight, health and have the best quality of life. I will dare you to do this simple challenge because I know you will feel a whole lot better. If you currently live a more active lifestyle you know what I am talking about.

Since the beginning of civilization until now, people have been looking for the magic pill or potion to bring them eternal youth, good health and a cure for all maladies. It is historically documented that, in the old ages, the pharaohs of Egypt and other kings and queens have embarked on the search for what is called "The Elixir Of Life" which would be a cure-all substance, a provider of good health and a substance, which would increase life expectancy. Instead, these endeavors led to inadvertent discoveries of some medicines that are still used today to treat a variety of diseases and ailments. These ancient medicinal discoveries eventually led the way to the evolving world of modern-day medicine.

Nowadays, as recent as 2006, this similar mentality regarding the search for "The Elixir of Life" is very much alive as I witness it daily in my pharmacy practice. Everybody is on the search for a pill or an "herb" or a "Natural drug" that will prevent disease that will prevent colds, give them "Energy" and that will make them slimmer. People at the pharmacy counter ask for pills that will "take away" their weight and health problems, that will bring them good health, boost their energy, and boost their immune systems while, at the same time, they go on consuming enormous amounts of "fattening foods" and go on leading totally inactive lifestyles.

Humans can never anticipate lifelong good health that comes by taking a pill. If there ever would be a panacea or a cure-all it would be this; "leading an **active** lifestyle." Lifelong good health, weight control, disease prevention or prevention of disease complications, are only the result of making favorable lifestyle choices regularly or most of the time. Most importantly we should lead an active lifestyle.

Leading an active lifestyle is one of only two ways we can control our weight and prevent muscle loss as we age. In correlation with active lifestyles, we must make balanced food choices. It is crucial to make these balanced food choices (as discussed above); also, when we choose to be sedentary, we can never avert disease and maintain our weight over the long haul, but weight and disease will creep up on us. If you choose to lead an active lifestyle and more than occasionally indulge, then you can still maintain your weight and prevent weight gain as well as prevent disease. This is not an encouragement to make less favorable food choices; in order for you to lose weight and maintain that loss, you have to make favorable choices in both your food and activity selections.

The Miraculous Benefits of an Active Lifestyle:

- Long-term weight control
- Long-term weight loss
- Increases fat loss even at rest
- Stress relief
- Reduces the pressure on your spine, bones, and joints
- Reduces joint and foot pain
- Reduces the incidents of arthritis
- Reduces the pressure and weight on the feet, consequently reducing foot discomfort and pain
- Reduces back pain
- Makes you feel good
- Is a sexual booster
- Drastically reduces erectile dysfunction problems
- Increases libido (sexual desires) in both men and women
- Wards off diseases
- Promotes regular bowels
- Promotes better sleep
- Decreases the incidence of depression or helps control it
- Decreases blood pressure
- Decreases cholesterol
- Increases good cholesterol
- Decreases the need for the number of medications and their doses for people who are diabetic and who take medications for diabetes, cholesterol and blood pressure
- Can revert heart disease, blood pressure, cholesterol problems and diabetes
- Keeps muscles inside our veins and arteries flexible, consequently preventing heart disease
- Thins the blood and prevents heart attacks as we age
- Increases muscle mass
- Prevents muscle loss due to aging and helps us stay independent as we age
- Improves the health of all humans regardless of age
- Helps us age gracefully
- Boosts our immune system and helps us fight infection and diseases and recover faster from them
- Maximizes weight loss from fat, even when we are at rest
- This is a Cure-All pill that everyone must have

Common Excuses Why People Choose to Remain Sedentary

Everyone should be asking the following question: "What makes me choose to be sedentary instead of trying to be active?" Here are some common excuses people come up with:

- "I don't have time" (This is the most common universal excuse that people have. They can sit and wait in the pharmacy waiting area for 45 minutes while waiting on their prescriptions).

- "It is hard. It takes a lot of effort."
- "Exercise is not for me."
- "I am not an athlete."

It is a misconception to think that people "have to exert too much effort" to get all of the health benefits from being active (including the benefits mentioned in the table above). If you will notice, the words in this guide are carefully chosen. If you look throughout this guide, you will not see the word "exercise" mentioned anywhere. I use the term "activity" because the word exercise alienates a lot of people. This word may have created a lot of misconceptions and myths. Some people think they have to go to the gym every day in order to get any health benefits.

Some people may not want to have the extra gym expense or may not have the time to go to the gym or do not know what to do in the gym once there. You don't have to go to the gym in order to increase your daily level of activity. But for your sake, do not remain sedentary and miss all the lifesaving benefits that an active lifestyle can bring to your life. Whatever excuse you might have, do not say that you "do not have time" to gain good health and spare yourself a heart attack. (See section "Tips to increase daily activity..." below.)

I have seen missed opportunities every day during my entire pharmacy career. The real life stories, in this guide, are key to my point. Numerous people that I have met through my pharmacy practice miss out on making good activity choices, and they mirror the staggering number of inactive people in the US. How many times have you gone to the pharmacy to drop off your prescriptions or to the doctor's office and you were told it was going to be a 20-30 minute wait; and you sat down in the waiting room that entire time. On your next doctor's visit, inform the attendant that you are in the hall walking and have her call you whenever it is your turn. This way, you will let off some steam from having to sit and wait for the doctor, and you'll get some exercise.

Next time you go to the pharmacy to get your prescriptions filled, you will not snap and flinch when a pharmacy staff member informs you it's going to be about 15-20 minutes to get your prescriptions filled. When we tell you it is going to be that long or longer, instead of sitting you might take a walk and not miss the opportunity to be active. Come to the pharmacy equipped with your rubber-padded comfortable shoes, and if your kids are with you, then it will be a family bonding time and all will go walking in and around the store. If the store is not big enough, go next door to a bigger store, outlet, strip mall or shopping center and do the walking. That is what an active lifestyle is all about. And that was your "gym trip" for the day. **You did not actually go to the gym; the gym is wherever you are, and wherever you choose to be.**

Choose to be active "now," instead of being sedentary, and cull all the benefits of an active lifestyle as detailed in the table above. Don't forget that an active lifestyle will boost your sexual life (see the section entitled "Boost Your Sexual Life").

How Anyone Can Make Over His or Her Current Sedentary Lifestyle And Make the Transition to an Active Lifestyle: Do It NOW and Permanently Lose 10 to 15 Pounds a Year

Choosing to have an active lifestyle is easier than you think. An active lifestyle means increasing the amount of moving around you do during any normal day; secondly, an active lifestyle means that you schedule, every other day, about 3-4 times a week, a sustained amount of activity for about 30-60 minutes in a progressive form which we will discuss further on in this guide. (These 30-45 minute bouts 3 to 4 times a week can actually be broken down into 2 or 3 10 or 15-minute bouts during the day.) This scheduled activity 3 or 4 times a week will not only give a boost to your weight loss, but it is also crucial in strengthening your heart and preventing heart disease.

Make Daily Choices to Increase Your Level of Activity

Increasing the amount of moving around during each day at a **brisk pace** (slightly faster than your normal pace) and depending less on automation is a major contributor to helping you burn more energy and lose weight. Increasing the amount of activity daily is as important as your diabetes medications in helping you control diabetes since activity causes your working muscles to need and take the sugar from your blood, consequently making your body less resistant to insulin. So activity helps make your insulin do its job better in reducing your blood sugar and makes your body more sensitive to its effects. That is almost how some of your oral diabetes medications work (See Action Step 2). Activity should go hand in hand with your diabetes medications and is an integral compliment to them in helping you bring diabetes under control.

Every move you make counts. You burn more energy when you stand than when you sit, and obviously, you also burn more energy when you walk than when you sit. You also burn more energy when you walk at a **brisk pace** than when you walk slowly. The most important task initially is to establish the habit of picking up more activity during the course of each day (refer to section that discusses how to start a good habit and to all the examples discussed there at the beginning of Action Step 4 and apply them here). Expect occasional forgetfulness at the beginning, such as forgetting to take the steps instead of the elevator; but forgive yourself and try to make a better choice next time.

Remember, you're trying to be more active only 80% of the time. Don't aim at perfection. **If you mess up here and there, try to do better the next time**. But whatever you do, do make another attempt and another one after that, in order to remain active during each and every day. After about 3 weeks or less of moving forward with these positive activity choices, you will automatically execute that activity without thinking of it.

Say you just decided, this minute, to start remembering to increase activity by parking your car far from the shopping center entrance. In the first 2-3 weeks, you might occasionally forget to park "further" and end up parking, habitually, in the very first spot. When you catch yourself doing that, if you still have not left the car, then back out and try to park in the very last spot or far away from the entrance of that shopping center. If you have already been in the store and you remembered that you should have parked far, let it go. Next time you come to that store or any other destination, make sure you remember to park further away. After 2-3 weeks of repeating this action, you will remember from the very first time to park further away, and you will actually "not want to" park close because it has become your new habit. You will be making that correct decision without hesitation anymore. Just like the parking brake story of that new car.

Those extra few trips with most of your daily choirs can get you to increase your walking by about 20 to 30 minutes daily. **This daily increase in your walking translates to a weight loss of about 10 to 15 pounds a year** depending on how much walking you average.

The Invaluable Use of a Pedometer

A good motivator to help you increase the amount of walking you do per day is to wear a pedometer. U.S. health organizations, including the American Diabetes Association, recommend **walking over 10,000 steps per day**. Buy that pedometer, set it up and get ready. When you wake up in the morning, wear the pedometer and set it to 0. You will see how motivating it is to make those extra steps in order to reach your goal. It is easily done. When afternoon arrives, and you are behind in your steps-taken goal, this will motivate you to take the extra steps and reach or exceed the 10,000 steps per day goal.

TIPS TO RAISE YOUR DAILY ACTIVITY LEVEL AT WORK, AT HOME AND WHILE SHOPPING

Always consult with your doctor before starting any activity. Remember to wear comfortable and rubber-padded shoes. Use common sense. If at times you are very busy then it is OK if you skip some trips or make them less frequently. If your work environment does not permit frequent trips, then cut back a little. **But one thing is for sure; no matter what work environment you are in, whether you work at home or commute to work, you can be a lot more active (at least 30 to 50% more) than you currently are by using some of these tips or by using your creativity and coming up with your own ideas for furthering your activity.**

- Walk around when you are on the phone. With corded phones, get a long extension and move 3-4 feet sideways. With cordless phones, you can move around the house and maybe move around outside the house.
- The 4-Foot rule (see below for details).
- Reduce TV watching and take the whole family on a 15-20 minute or longer power walk. If time does not allow, you can do a couple of bouts of 15 minute activity per day, before your lunch break and right after work.
- Make frequent trips to put several objects away or to move objects from point A to point B.
- You can do slow jumps in place while raising your hands to the side or do any activity in place, even when you're watching TV at home. You can do it alone or you can do it with a friend or your spouse or significant other.

- Make small additional walking efforts (30-45 seconds) with every or most chore during the day, at the supermarket, or while doing any kind of shopping. This adds up to big rewards and results at the end of each day, each month, and each year.
- Do not use drive-throughs ANYWHERE. Park your car at the last spot in the parking lot of that restaurant.
- Volunteer to do the walking chores of others.
- At home or at work, sip on water but fill your cup half way and make more frequent trips to refill it up.
- Use smaller garbage bags at home and make more frequent trips to the dumpster, dumping each small bag at a time.

- Use the stairs instead of the elevator.
- Buy a stationary bicycle, an elliptical machine or treadmill according to what you can afford, and do about 20 minutes in front of the TV daily, or 3-5 times a week.
- Walk in the mall or the local Wal-Mart.
- Walk while waiting at the doctor's office or waiting for your prescriptions,
- Make more frequent trips to set up the dining table and then to take dirty plates, utensils and pans back to the kitchen.
- Do not delegate any task requiring movement to anyone else. Use the 3 or 4 step rule when you are at your desk at work or home.
- Make frequent trips to the basement to get several items, making one trip for each item.
- In the shopping mall, take the chance to do more walking.
- At your desk, use a manual stapler instead of an electric effortless stapler.
- Use a manual pencil sharpener instead of an electric and effortless sharpener.
- Use a manual can opener instead of using the electric one.
- Take a 30-minute brisk walk outdoors.
- Do your own housecleaning.
- Do your own yard work.
- Use your creativity and come up with your own ideas in your own environment.

The 4-Foot Rule

While at your desk or place of work, place all the tools that you use during your workday within a 3 to 4 feet radius from you and **not** within an arm's reach from your current position. For example, put the stapler and the paper clips at the end of one side of your desk, then the penholder and the phone on the opposite side. Keep the trash can about 4 feet away from you. Every time you need to use frequently used items, you would have to get up and take a few steps, making the extra effort of walking without causing any loss of work productivity. (Reminder: wear comfortable rubber-padded shoes to prevent the extra impact on your knees and joints).

The Crucial Importance of Scheduling about 30 Minutes Of Brisk Walking 3-5 Times a Week

Before starting any activity, consult with your doctor to get clearance. Scheduling as little as 30 minutes of activity (such as walking, swimming, cycling. See a detailed list below of similar activities) 3 times a week, at a brisk pace (a speed slightly faster than your normal pace), in addition to the increased activity during each day, will help you boost your weight loss due to fat burning; this will also help you control diabetes, help you reduce stress, reduce cholesterol, blood pressure and **most importantly, it is the only way to help you strengthen your heart muscle.**

In order to derive major health benefits, you do not have to go to the gym for 2 hours. You surely can find 30 minutes every other day, or about two bouts of 15 minutes of walking daily most days of the week. When you are scheduling those 30-60 minutes of continuous walking several days a week, you maximize fat loss.

What other choices besides walking can generate similar results? Any activity of your choice that gets you moving in a steady uninterrupted pace for 30 minutes or two 15-minute bouts that you consider fun, such as:

- Cycling indoors (on a stationary bicycle) or outdoors
- Walking on a treadmill
- Walking around the house
- Walking in a shopping center or outdoors
- Jumping in place with side arm movements at home while watching your favorite show
- Swimming (ideal for diabetics with leg pain)
- Pool aerobics or pool exercises (ideal for diabetics with leg pain or neuropathy)

If you have access to a gym, then all the elliptical machines, treadmills, cycling machines, and stair-steppers can also be used for variety.

Is 30 Minutes Every Other Day Enough?

Yes. You can remain at 30 minutes, 3-4 times a week, if you wish and still get all the miraculous health benefits of activity. However, if you gradually (read next section to know what progressive or gradual means) increase your speed or time, up to 45-60 minutes to about 4 or 5 times a week, then you will have a solid edge over weight loss.

What Is a Reasonable Approach to Progression in the Amount and Duration of the Activity You Choose?

The first 2-3 weeks, you are establishing a habit foundation, so the most important task initially is to incorporate activity in your lifestyle by starting with 30 minutes every other day. Do not skip that scheduled session, but plan your social life around it. You are not only establishing a habit foundation for life, but also your body muscles, joints, and ligaments will get stronger and become ready for more actions. If you go too fast too soon, then you increase the risk of injury to those muscles and ligaments, and you may lose weight from unwanted places such as your muscles, while losing less fat than you want. After 3-4 weeks of performing that scheduled activity of your choice for about 30 minutes every other day, then you can increase each session by 10 minutes per week per session up to one hour per session as follows:

Week	Activity
1, 2 & 3	30 minutes of brisk walking, cycling, or any activity you choose every other day (make a different activity choice periodically)
4	40 minutes every other day
5	40-50 minutes 4 times a week
6	45-60 minutes 4 times a week (add a twist by including hilly terrain or including inclination on your treadmill or on your exercise machine)
7	45-60 minutes 5 times a week

Maintain, thereafter, with 45-60 minutes per day, about 4-5 times a week. Should you desire to go back to 3 times a week then you are in control with all the variables and you will **always** get health benefits from an active lifestyle.

Warm Up and Cool Down

For health and safety purposes and for injury prevention, any time you get involved in a continuous type of activity always start and end your activity with a slow, 5-minute movement.

For the curious only:

The Benefits of the 5-Minute Warm-Up at the Beginning Of Your Chosen Activity

Warm-up is intended to raise your body temperature slowly, and by doing so, warms your muscles and joints and ligaments and prepares them for action. Muscles and joints that are warm are less likely to be injured and can generate more power.

- The initial slow movement helps your brain gradually release nerve substances to prepare your heart, lungs, and muscles for the upcoming activity.

- The initial slow movement warm-up session helps you detect any pain or discomfort to any parts of your body and make adjustments accordingly. You should decide to not go through with activity if in discomfort. If at the start of the warm-up session or any time during that activity, you feel nauseated, dizzy or drowsy, then you should make the decision to stop that training session and seek medical advice. Check your blood sugar since your blood sugar maybe dropping too low; due to the effect of the activity you are doing and your diabetes medications.

The Benefit of the Last 5-Minute Cool Down Period

The gradual reduction of speed at the end of your session instead of an abrupt stop will help you do the following:

- Gradually reduce the amount of nerve substances that has been released into your body during that bout of activity. If you get into the habit of stopping abruptly after a moderately intense session of walking or cycling or light jogging, then that may cause irregular heartbeats.
- Cooling down at the end of the session helps you ease out of that session and relax your working muscles and body gradually. You will feel better.

How Fast Should You Go During that Scheduled Activity? The "Talk Test"

The speed should be brisk, faster than your normal pace. Whether you are walking, cycling or performing any other similar activity, a good way to gauge whether the speed is good enough for favorable weight loss results and health benefits is "The Talk Test." Let's say you decided to go for a 30-minute walk with a partner. So you start:

1. First, the slow pace 5-minute warm-up of whatever activity you choose.

2. The next 20 minutes, increase your speed to where you can barely complete a full sentence without gasping for air. If you try to say one or two words and you are gasping for air, then your intensity is too high. Drop your speed slightly or stop the movement of your arms periodically until you are able to talk comfortably (4-5) words in a sentence without having to gasp.

3. On the other hand, if you are saying 2-3 sentences and laughing before you are gasping for air, then you probably are taking a slow stroll or still in the warm-up phase. Pick up your speed and start moving your arms at your

sides, rhythmically, until you are able to say 4-5 words comfortably without having to gasp for air.

INTERVAL MOVEMENT CYCLES: A MAJOR POWERFUL WEIGHT-LOSS BOOSTER

This principal offers an efficient technique that anybody at any level of fitness, from completely sedentary to the most advanced, can use it. In a speedy way, it helps you:

1. Become more efficient at burning fat.
2. Lose weight more quickly and steadily (when varying the intensity periodically and at your convenience).
3. Strengthen your heart.

After the first 5-minutes of warm-up, you will start a cycle of fast and slow-paced movements as follows:

1. At the end of the warm-up period, pick up the speed to near maximum (but not quite maximum) of your comfort level for about 45 seconds (you have to time it with your stop watch).
2. Then drop the speed to a brisk pace (not the warm-up speed) for 5 minutes. Then pick up again for 45 seconds, and then slow down for 5 minutes, going back and forth up to a total of 20 minutes.
3. The last 5 minutes: Reduce your speed to a slow cool-down and relaxing end.

HOW YOU CAN VARY THE TWIST

The following week you increase the fast cycle phase of that interval by 30 seconds to achieve a 1 minute and 15 second bout, and you drop the slower walking cycle by 30 seconds to 4 minutes and 30 seconds, while keeping all else the same, meaning the same amount of cooling down and warming up, and the same total 30 minutes for that week as in the progression schedule. The week after, you bump up another 30 seconds for the fast phase, and you drop the slow down period by 30 seconds. If it is a week when you are doing the activity for 45 minutes, then the first and last 5 minutes always remain slow; and in-between, you alternate the fast and slow interval cycles. If you choose to become more advanced (you don't have to) several weeks later (and not before), then the fast cycle may become 3 or 4 minutes and the slow phase may be dropped to 2 or 3 minutes.

The Revealing Benefits of Choosing One Progression Criteria at a Time

A good word of advice as you are progressing: take a gradual and a balanced approach. Don't get overenthusiastic, skip the progression model we discussed above; if you start increasing your walking time by 30 minutes every other workout, and increasing the intervals to a 5-minute faster cycle and 2-minute slower cycle by the second week, then this is a formula for disaster and for inevitable injury. After you have been sedentary, your heart, lungs, muscles, energy system, joints, ligaments, and just about everything in your body need about 3-4 weeks of adequately spaced workouts and rest phases to progress to a minimum foundation level. Only then can you gradually progress to your desired goal and speed. Any progress needs to be achieved in small increments and over a period of time, usually a week, before physical improvements occur.

For instance, if you are currently walking 3 times a week for a total of 20 minutes, and you have a goal to increase your walking bouts to about 45 minutes each time, raising the frequency to about 5 times a week and including hilly terrains and you start performing all of these 3 tasks as of the following week, then your injury risk becomes too high, and you start actually losing muscle mass more than fat, since your energy utilization system has not become efficient.

Your brain will start telling you that what you are doing is perceived as a major change from your usual behavior (of the previous week), and gets you to reject the activity and quit. As mentioned earlier, your risk of injury becomes much higher, and when you injure a muscle or a ligament due to this faulty action, then part of your recovery is to be off for several weeks. You will have actually defeated yourself by not being able to perform any activity due to your injury. The idea is to start a progression plan and make your body progress and avoid injury. Choose only one progression criteria at a time, as indicated in the progression plan above.

What Time of Day Is Best for Your Chosen Activity?

There is not one particular time of day, for activity, which gives you better results. However, choose the time of day, make it to your liking or whenever you feel you have the most energy. Some people are morning people: if you are a morning person and wish to perform that activity in the morning, go ahead and do so. Some others prefer to perform it in the evening, after work. Choose your preferred activity and preferred time. One thing you do not have to do, though, if you are not a morning person, don't get up at 4:00 a.m. and head to the gym and stay there for 2 hours. Remember, this is not a balanced approach, and by waking up earlier, you are putting more strain and stress on yourself. Choose a time that's good for you; but whatever you do, don't skip your workout, and work your social life around it.

You are in total control of all the variables. Always remain flexible, and you don't "always" have to progress. You might reach a comfort level with your lifestyle, and you just want to maintain what you have been doing. If one week you performed only two scheduled walking sessions and you have been less active daily during that week, it is okay. Go easy on yourself, and remember to always adopt a balanced approach. The key issue here is to include a variety in whatever you do to keep your gains growing. Remember, the gains don't always come from doing more and by increasing your workout time or load. The gains will come if you remain persistent in your actions. Always go for variety, do something different every week. That will also keep your mind and muscles from adapting to being exposed to the same thing and will boost your body to give you better weight loss results and better control of your disease condition.

ESTABLISH ACTIVITY HABIT PATTERNS THROUGH PERSISTENT ACTION

When you're trying to establish new favorable habits, remember you have to repeat those actions several times a week (after about 3 weeks or so, they will have become a habit). In this case, if you're trying to establish the habit of walking 30-45 minutes 3-4 times a week, then you need to repeat that action, and you need to schedule all your other social activities around this action, and do not skip it. For instance, say it is Wednesday, and it is 6:00 p.m., and you just got home from work, and you had scheduled 30 minutes of stationary cycling in front of your TV before having supper. As soon as you walk in the door, your neighbor calls and says she is bringing the kids over and coming in for a visit. Now you are faced with a choice to make. First, either respond to her with a "Yes" and skip what is going to be something that will make you feel good and will relieve your stress. or tell her "no" and refuse skipping that activity; tell your neighbor to come a little bit later or join you with your activity.

Say you choose the latter, and you tell your neighbor you are about to start riding your stationary bike and that you prefer she stop by after you are done. Now your neighbor is wondering why she doesn't do the same. Better yet, suggest to your neighbor to join you for a 30-minute walk around the block, or you can do the walk at the mall. You can come up with a number of creative ideas.

The Feeling-Good Factor

After 3-4 weeks of persistently repeating actions and establishing your new habit of becoming more active, you will start enjoying and feeling the pleasure of what you are doing and experiencing the stress relief. This will be your healing time from outside stresses, and it will be that special private time for you. During (and at the end of) each scheduled activity bout, you will feel you have been cleansed of your worries. Your weight loss results will have been compounding, and you will feel relieved and healed emotionally and physically. You will also feel a sense of pride and experience an overall sense of "feeling good" and accomplishment. As time goes by, and you keep at it, the benefit to your health, body, and mind will be invaluable, incredibly rewarding, and keep on compounding.

Why Is It Essential to Include Variety In Your Chosen Activities?

- To relieve boredom from a set routine.
- To keep your sessions stimulating and get you to look forward to your next one.
- One of the most crucial reasons to include a variety in your activity is that your brain will get your body to adapt to whatever action you are doing. Then your weight loss progress may slow down unless, periodically, you add a variety factor and you change one thing at a time as mentioned above, such as including hilly terrain and changing the type of activity you are doing. For example, if you were cycling around the block, then you can do stationary cycling as a change, or you can walk at the park, or increase the time of your walking activity by say only 10 minutes for the next few sessions, etc.

The Fun Factor

Don't forget to keep the activity fun and interesting. Choose only an activity that you personally favor and enjoy.

You are in control of all the variables; use them in a balanced manner to your advantage and to suit your lifestyle. For example, say you were sedentary and you lately increased the amount of walking during the day, and you have scheduled 20 minutes of brisk walking 3 times a week. You will notice, initially, a little discomfort and a sense that things are "different." But after 3-4 weeks of repeating the planned walking activity, you will feel that everything has become easier and that you are not expanding "as much effort" for the same activity.

Your body has adapted to the load of activity you were performing. You will still gain the same health benefits if you keep everything else the same. However, if you add a small twist or a variety to what you are doing, you will boost your weight loss further and keep your body geared to culling better results.

So what variables can you use? The variables don't always have to be more strenuous or more time-consuming; they just have to be different. These variables can be used on various days and you get to make the decision of what variable you employ and for how long and when.

A Variety of Activity Choices to Include in Your Scheduled Activity Session on Different Days

After the 5-minute warm-up, you can choose either of the following:

- Use interval cycles during walking, cycling or any other activity you choose.
- Use steady walking at a brisk pace the whole time between warm-up and cool-down for all training sessions for a whole week.
- Choose hilly terrains (Tip: When you are walking an ascending slope, slow down your speed a little).
- Use side-rhythmic-arm movement along with walking.
- Choose a slightly more intense interval activity, such as a 2-minute light jog or speed walking for your "quick-paced activity," and a 2-minute brisk walk for the slightly "slower- paced activity."
- The following week, choose a total of 50 minute of steady brisk walking each scheduled day for the whole week. If you have access to a gym where you can find treadmills, cycling, and elliptical machines, then use a different program intensity at times, and at other times, use a totally different machine. If one day, you elect to use a cycling machine, then two workouts later, you can choose to work out on the elliptical machine or the stepper. At other times, you can choose to use 3 different machines for 15-minute intervals each during the same session. You can choose any combination according to your likes and dislikes.

- You can choose 1 whole week of in-place fast walking or light jogging with lateral arm movement (and you can do this in front of your TV, while watching a movie of your choice).

- If you have access to a gym and to all the machines listed above, you can choose a different inclination and a different duration time for your session. For instance, one day you can do a total of 40 minutes; the next scheduled session you can do a total of 50 minutes. The next scheduled session you can do a total of 35 minutes, any combination that you desire.

- You can alternate between using machines (if you have access to them) on one day during that week, and on the next scheduled session you can choose a non-machine-type activity, such as brisk walking and alternating lateral arm rises while walking. The following scheduled session, you can use your bicycle for a total 50-minute-ride one day, or you can do a 35-50 minute swimming session or in-water activity, if you have access to a swimming pool.

- You can use any combination of the above. Allow your mind to fire up with creativity, but always stick with the basic guidelines as recommended in "Always Stick to the Basics" (the next section).

PS: Keep it varied. Variety boosts further health benefits and further weight loss beyond a plateau (a plateau is when you reach a point when you are no longer loosing weight and your progress is no longer improving).

Always Stick to the Basics

Whatever activity you decide to choose, always stay within the basic guidelines of each session:

- Have a 5-minute warm-up and cool-down session.
- Use the talk test to gauge your intensity (see details about the talk test in "How fast should you go...?" above.
- Stick to a total activity time of 30-60 minutes for each scheduled session and do this between 3-5 times per week. Occasionally, if you wish, you can move up to 90 minutes, but not less than 8 weeks after you started working out.
- Progress gradually, in small, increments once a week.
- Always aim at balance in your lifestyle, practicing what has been discussed, most of the time; allow yourself to break the rules sometimes. Be flexible, and do not be locked into rigid expectations.
- Come up with your own creative ideas that work for you and your lifestyle, and remember that you are in control.

- **The importance of rest:** Rest and having about 8 hours of sleep daily are as important as activity. The reason you schedule activity every other day is to give time to your body on that day off to recuperate and be ready for the next session. A rested body and muscles will provide you with results you desire. Doing too much and overdoing beyond the progression plan described above is counterproductive and provide you with opposite results.
- *Be flexible* in your choices but remain persistent. If occasionally you had a busy week, and then you can only schedule activity once, then that's fine. Balance out that action by increasing your daily activity at work for that week. or occasionally you came home and did not feel like going through with that scheduled activity, then lie off and take a break. **But be persistent and pick up that scheduled activity of your choice the following week or next time.** *It is only with your persistent actions and favorable choices most of the times that you can have a lifelong good health and permanent favorable results.*

What About Jogging, Racquetball, Intensive Training And Team Sports?

Nobody has to jog in order to achieve health benefits or lose weight. In fact, if you have been sedentary, it is not recommended that you jog (initially) or be involved in intense training. If you have been sedentary, and you start engaging in highly intense activity, such as jogging or racquetball, early on in the first 2-3 weeks, then you may tend to lose some muscle mass more than fat weight. This is not what you want. You are trying to lose weight mostly from the fat deposits.

Instead, you could use a powerful technique referred to as "Interval Cycles" as discussed above. As you become more fit, and after at least 3-4 weeks of persistent scheduled activity, your body structure has then evolved and improved and your heart has become more adept; in addition, your energy system has become more advanced at breaking down your fat and using it as energy; it is "only at this point" that you can choose to engage in such intensive activities. When you are less fit, high-impact sports can possibly trigger heart problems.

As for team sports such as football, basketball, baseball, tennis, or volleyball, the limitation here would be not finding steady partners to play with, and also, these can be time-consuming sessions. Team sports can be performed during weekends as a pastime. But weekend activities alone cannot build good health, a strong heart, nor can they be depended upon for weight loss. Only steady activity daily throughout the full week, can give you the results you are looking for.

Activity Log

It is a great idea to keep track of the amount of activity you do daily, at least for the first few weeks, until you have a feel of the amount of activity you should be up to daily. It is also a visual motivator to see your steps build up to over 10,000 steps daily and to monitor your sugar levels and see those levels drop before your eyes on the monitor. So get that pedometer and start logging your daily activity. See a blank sample of the Activity Log at the end of this guide. You may copy the blank activity log as frequently as you need to.

Safety Tips

- Consult with your doctor before starting any activity and get clearance to begin.
- Lay off from any activity and have complete rest when you are under any sort of trauma or illness, and consult with your doctor on when you can resume activity if you have any of the following: colds and respiratory infections, fever, dizziness, any kind of pain or discomfort (including chest pain), or whenever you don't feel up to par or when you have difficulty breathing.

Proper Gear for Your Activity Sessions

Here are some suggestions about what to wear during cold and warm weather, and what important tools you need on the way to your active lifestyle.

Footwear

Wear rubber-padded comfortable shoes (if the shoes are new, break them in gradually, 2-3 hours a day for a couple of weeks). Rubber-padded shoes can be the usual tennis shoes or rubber-padded walking shoes. Nowadays, you have stylish shoes that have rubber padding on the bottom and are ideal for work. If, for cosmetic reasons, you don't want to wear tennis shoes, you can take these comfortable padded shoes or tennis shoes along with you to work, and there you can change into your more comfortable shoes. Always wear rubber-padded comfortable shoes anywhere you go, even at work, so you can remain active at all times. Importantly, rubber-padded shoes will lessen the impact on your joints and ligaments and will reduce the stress that is placed on them.

Pedometer

- The price of an average good pedometer should be somewhere between $15 and $18.
- As soon as you buy the pedometer, set it up with your own criteria. Follow the instructions on the package.
- Reset to 0 steps every morning and aim, gradually, at reaching over 10,000 steps daily (as recommended by the American Heart and American Diabetes Association).
- Wear the pedometer correctly, horizontally on your waist (belt or pants). The cover of that pedometer must be shut. Otherwise, the pedometer will not function properly and will not log your steps.

Stopwatch

It is important to own an inexpensive stopwatch in order to monitor your activity time and your interval cycles. An average price of a good stopwatch should be between $10 and $15.

Clothing for Various Climates

<u>Warm Weather</u>: Wear 100% cotton walking shorts and t-shirts, as cotton is the most absorbent.

<u>Cold Weather</u>: If you choose outdoor activities during cold weather, then dress in layers in order to prevent heat loss from your body. Cover your head with a hood or a cap to prevent heat being lost through the top of your head. Keep your muscles warm.

The Importance of Water Replenishment and Hydration

- Water is the most important nutrient.
- You need to have 6-8 glasses of water per day.
- Also drink before, during and after scheduled activity in addition to your 8 daily glasses of water.

- Drink cold water in warm weather, as it cools high internal body temperatures; and cold water is absorbed faster than room-temperature water when the body is hot.
- Water is essential for life, as over 70% of the body is made of water.
- Adequate water intake will keep your bowels regular.
- Just about every process in the body, including energy breakdown, requires the presence of water.
- Adequate water intake keeps the kidneys and the entire body functioning properly, and it keeps your skin well hydrated.

Tips on Staying Active while Having Physical Challenges and Leg Neuropathic Pain

If you have pain in your feet or any other part of your legs, then let the pain and discomfort be your guide by stopping when discomfort sets in. But that does not give you an excuse to remain sedentary all hours of the day. *Here are some activity tips*:

- Wear comfortable rubber (broken-in) padded shoes.
- Walk for bouts of 5-10 minutes or until pain or discomfort arrives.
- At home or at work, do frequent getting up and walking around and doing your own chores and trips; don't delegate them to anyone. In other words, if you're sitting in the living room and you feel like having a glass of water, don't wait until your spouse or your children pass by to tell them to get you the glass of water. You get up and get it. That's not going to cause your legs to hurt tremendously if you do that 30 second or 45 second bout of activity. If you're preparing supper or lunch and you're trying to take a bunch of stuff to the kitchen table, try to make frequent trips from the kitchen to the dining table, taking each item, one at a time, and you're achieving some activity in your back and forth trips; make this attempt at extra activity when you're starting the meal and when you're completing it.
- Use non-weight bearing movements (such as swimming pool activities, moving around in a swimming pool) or you can use stationary cycling or elliptical machines if you have access to any of them.
- Frequent getting-up and moving-around movements will help you burn more energy and will help sensitize your body and prepare it to respond more positively to the effects of insulin.
- You can also perform the rubber tubing exercises that have been mentioned previously.

IF YOU ARE IN A WHEELCHAIR:

- Strengthen your arms and shoulders by pushing your own wheels periodically during the day during 10-15 minute bouts; do this daily. Working your upper body muscles will help you become stronger, more independent and help control your diabetes by getting your muscles to take in the sugar from your blood and help your body to be sensitive to the effects of insulin.
- If you're confined to a wheelchair and you can still do upper body movement, you can use your arms, which allows you to be able to do the rubber tubing activities that have been mentioned in the previous section.

Actually, it is very crucial to keep your upper body muscles and arm muscles strong, in order to be able to perform various daily tasks. It is absolutely crucial to keep your body muscles toned and to keep your heart and lungs functioning properly by remaining active. The longer you remain sedentary, the faster you lose these capacities, and the worse your condition becomes. Remember, movement and activity is one of the best medicines. You need to perform any activity with the capacity that you have; let your pain and discomfort be your guide in when you should stop, but take every opportunity that you have to create any kind of motion during each hour of each day, using your upper body.

What to Remember from All the Prior Information In This Activity Section

What is essential for you to remember from this whole activity section is that activity performed persistently daily and weekly helps you in:

- Losing weight
- Maintaining weight loss permanently
- Achieving all types of health benefits (see the section entitled "The Miraculous Benefits of an Active Lifestyle")
- Preventing disease and disease complications

HOW TO ADOPT AN ACTIVE LIFESTYLE:

1. Increase the amount of daily walking you do at home, at work, while shopping or any other chance you have.

2. Schedule continuous 30 minute walking bouts (or two 15-minute bouts) 3 times a week (see the section entitled "Scheduling 30 Minutes of Brisk Walking").

3. Work your body muscles for 15-20 minutes once or twice a week.

4. Adopt a gradual progression approach by choosing one progression criteria each week, one at a time. (See the section entitled "Choose One Progression Criteria Each Week at a Time").

5. Adopt a "variety" approach in order to boost and expedite your progress. (See the section entitled "Boost Your Progress With Variety").

6. Get enough rest and about 7-8 hours of sleep daily.

7. Don't forget to reward yourself because you have earned it.

8. Finally, don't forget to drink 6-8 glasses of water daily and before and during every activity session.

Permanent Weight Loss

Do We Burn More Calories at Rest or When We Move Around?

Actually, **up to** a staggering 75% of the total energy that humans expand or burn during each day happens at rest. Probably you have read or heard of the term "Basic Metabolic Rate" or in short, "BMR." This is referred to the amount of energy or calories your body needs to keep you alive and keep your internal body organs (such as muscles, brain, heart, lungs, kidneys, liver, skin, tissue and all other body processes) working and functioning continuously with or without our conscious effort. On top of that, **up to** an additional 10% of our total daily energy expanded is used to metabolize the food we eat. This translates to a final tally of up to a whopping 85% of the total calories you burn during any given day, while sleeping, while resting, and while you are digesting your food and without your conscious effort.

People who are overweight and are leading sedentary lifestyles burn a lower percentage of energy at rest (lower than the normal 85%). Those "less active people" probably burn closer to no more than 50 or 60% of energy at rest. However, their counterparts, the active people who have made favorable lifestyle choices and who choose to continually lead an active lifestyle as well as make balanced food choices and increase their high-fiber food intake (such as whole grain and oat bran) actually boost their body burning capacity to a maximum of 85%.

Is this amazing or what? Let's say, at any given day, you burn a total of 1800 calories, and of those, your body can burn up to 1500 calories while at rest and while metabolizing the food you eat. The remaining calories you will burn during the day while moving around, whether at the office or while shopping or performing any other activity-based task.

Can Anyone Manipulate Their Body's Capacity to Burn Maximum Energy and Lose Weight while at Rest?

Of course, all of us can. Here are some ways you can start boosting your BMR or your body's capacity to burn more calories at rest and lose more weight while sleeping or during any other time:

1. Increase the amount of activity and walking during each day as described before, especially during your scheduled activities (especially when including "Interval Movement Cycles" as described above. This is a powerful technique to boost BMR) during each week. Activity not only helps you burn calories during the time that you are doing them, but also for several hours after you stop. The more you engage in activity and become more advanced, the more your body becomes efficient at burning more fuel for several hours after you stop that activity.

2. Maintaining and increasing your very precious muscle mass is hugely important; by increasing or maintaining your muscle mass, your body burns more calories at rest to keep your muscle cells alive. The more muscle you lose (whether from inactivity or quick weight loss from dieting) the fewer calories you burn. One of the main reasons people gain weight as they age, even if their food consumption has not changed or increased, is muscle loss.

3. Don't ever diet again. Losing weight quickly, through dieting, is a main reason for fast muscle loss. Consequently, less energy is burned at rest to preserve the muscle that has been lost. As a result, fat accumulates much more easily.

4. Don't skip meals or snacks. You boost your body's capacity to burn calories at rest by consuming 3 main meals and 2 fruit snacks. More importantly, when you get into the habit of making food choices that are high in fiber (from List A), such as consuming whole grain, oat bran products, beans and bean products, vegetables, fruits as discussed in the food section, you will boost your body's capacity to burn more energy and calories to metabolize these high fiber foods. You lose weight in the process! Don't forget that **you burn an additional 250 calories per day by consuming about 35gm of fiber daily (This is a powerful but simple tool in your hand).**

5. Get a good 8 hours of sleep. While sleeping, your body spends an enormous amount of energy replenishing nutrients and keeping all your internal body organs working properly. Whenever we get less than 8 hours of sleep, the less energy we burn.

These favorable lifestyle choices will be a boost to your capacity to burn calories while at rest and while digesting food. **Anyone can tap into this enormous weight loss powerhouse called Basic Metabolic Rate.**

Quick Tips on How Anyone Can Start Immediately Losing Weight and Keep It Off for Life

How Can Anyone Shave Off 250 to 300 Calories Or More Daily from Food?

You will lose about 1-2 pounds per week by creating a total deficit of about 500-700 calories per day between the total amount of food consumed and the amount of walking and the total daily energy burnt or expanded. How you can do that? You can at least shave off about 250 to 300 calories daily, **simply,** when you choose a high fiber cereal for breakfast, and for both lunch and dinner you stick 80% of time with food choices from List A to fill an imaginary average round size dinner plate as discussed in the "Meal Blueprint" in the "Food" section Above (Half the plate with veggies, a quarter the meat and a quarter the high fiber carbs).

Also when you consume those 2 fruit snacks daily instead of dense and heavy snacks from vending machines at work, it will contribute to shaving off unwanted calories. By far the major contributor to shaving off additional calories is the switch from regular soft drink to a diet one or water. Don't forget that **increasing your total daily fiber consumption up to 35 gm will get you to burn an additional 250 calories**. This is easily done; refer to the section titled " How to get 35gm of fiber daily and loose an additional 250 calories daily," in the discussion about "Carbohydrates" before the "Meal Blueprint" section.

How Can Anyone Increase Their Energy Burning (Expansion) By 250 to 300 Calories?

Anyone can expand energy by doing more daily walking at work, home or while shopping and by scheduling an additional 30 to 45 minutes 3 to 5 times weekly (for heart benefits and general health maintenance benefits) as discussed in detail in the "Activity" section above.

Undoubtedly anybody can create an energy deficit of about 500 to 700 calories daily and lose an average of 1 to 2 pounds weekly without "Dieting" and without setting foot in the gym.

Simple Tips for Immediate Weight loss
(Results Start within Days)

At the start of any favorable actions for weight loss goals it will take several days from the start of those efforts before weight loss starts to occur. Remember that you are not aiming to lose weight now and regain it in 6 months but you want a permanent weight loss. So your efforts need to be *persistent* and *balanced* in order to achieve this endeavor. Here is a summary of what we just discussed about losing 1 to 2 pounds a week and keep it off permanently (the followings are estimates):

Favorable Choice	Weight Loss Per Week
• Consume 35 grams of fiber per day (see List A for food with higher fiber content. Also see discussion about high fiber carbs and how you can easily get 35gm of fiber in the Carbohydrates discussion before the "Meal Blueprint" section.	.50 pounds per week
• Switch from sugar-laden soft drinks and juices to diet soft drinks, flavored water with no calories, or iced tea (sweetened with artificial sweeteners).	.75 pounds per week
• Snack on fruits and vegetables instead of chips, pretzels, packaged snacks that are laden with sugar and salts (from vending machines).	.25 pounds per week
• Reduce portion sizes.	.25 to .50 pounds per week
• Increase the amount of walking you do by only 20 minutes throughout each day while at work, home, shopping, or doing any other daily chores as discussed in the activity section.	.25 to .50 pounds per week
• Schedule activity of 30-60 minutes of brisk walking 3-5 times a week as discussed in the activity section.	.50 pounds per week
Estimated Weekly Weight Loss:	**About 1-3 pounds per week**

"I Don't Know Why I Am Not Losing Weight" (Troubleshooting)

Here could be some reasons why you are not losing much weight. You must be either underestimating the amount and types of food you are eating (thus consuming more than what your body expands or burns) and/or overestimating the amount of activity you are doing. Account for everything that goes in your mouth. Get in the habit, initially, of recording your daily food consumption on the daily log I provided you at the end of the guide.

You might want a snack mid afternoon, so you buy a medium size bag of chips (an item in the less favorable carbs in List B) and you eat the whole thing. You do this every day. Instead, a more balanced approach would be to have some mixed nuts (a half palm-full) plus a fruit of your choice, most days of the week. Once or twice that week you limit yourself to a small bag of baked chips or some whole grain crackers (Triscuits made with whole grain) with a piece of cheese.

You could also be thinking, "I am just in the mood for some coffee." So you go and buy yourself a "small" "Frappucino" that has loads of sugar, which contributes to weight gain. Instead, you might get a cup of coffee and use a sweetener to sweeten it. or you might say, "I'm just having some cheese" and when you evaluate the portion size objectively that "some cheese" turns out to be half a block or more per day.

You also might think you are active during the day by doing "a lot of walking" at work, but actually you might not be doing enough (You underestimate your activity level). The best visual motivator is a pedometer; aiming, gradually, at walking over 10,000 steps daily, as discussed in the activity section. When you weigh yourself once a week, you can assess your success and make minor changes immediately, taking appropriate actions in a quick fashion.

WHEN YOU ARE NOT GETTING THE REASONABLE WEIGHT LOSS RESULTS YOU WANT

All of us have a tendency to slip back to old eating or unfavorable lifestyle habits, but like anything else, the more you practice making better food and lifestyle choices the better you get at it. Remember that **mastering a task is not an on/off switch but it is a**

Lifestyle Choices

process. When you are not getting the weight loss results you want, then ask yourself these questions and rectify the situation quickly by referring to the appropriate section in this guide:

- "Am I moving and walking enough past 10,000 steps daily?" or "have I been sitting more in front of the TV and moving less?" If not then reverse this and refer to the "Activity" section above and **practice** the tips provided to increase activity daily.

- Walk while waiting for anything instead of sitting. Anytime anybody asks you to "have a seat and wait" for "your turn to see the Dr." "for your prescriptions to be filled" etc…, then tell them "Oh no, I will be walking around until you call me." Don't miss a great opportunity to get walking while waiting for an appointment, or while filling your gas tank or other opportunities as are presented to you. So get moving.

- "Am I eating enough fiber?" If not then reverse your action by raising daily fiber as discussed in the "Food" section. Please refer to that section for further details on the benefits of fiber and it's weight loss boosting effect,

- "Have I been skipping meals or snacks?" Skipping meals is an action that contributes tremendously to weight gain. Refer to the "Meal Blueprint" in the Food section for a balanced meal distribution throughout the day.

- "What have I been eating for snacks?" Have you been forgetting to bring fruit to work and have been snacking more on dense packaged salty or sweet snacks, most of the time, that are void of nutrients and do nothing but contribute to weight gain? If so, then bring to work snacks from the fruits and "Snacks" sections in List A as suggested by the "Meal Blueprint."

- "Have my portion sizes gradually become bigger?" If so, reduce them again to a balanced amount to match that imaginary average round size plate in the distribution as discussed in the "Meal Blueprint."

- "Have I been making food choices more frequently from List B (less favorable and contribute to weight gain) rather than List A (more favorable, help prevent disease and contribute to weight loss)?" If so reverse this trend and refer to those lists provided in the "Food" section above.

- "Have I been drinking regular soft drinks and fruit juices more regularly now and returned to sweetening my coffee and tea with mega amounts of sugar?" Sugar in soft drinks and all the other drinks is a major contributor to obesity. Make drink choices from List A such as water, diet soft drinks (limit to 1 or 2 per day), and sweeten your drinks with Splenda.

- "Have I been duplicating food choices from the same food groups with every meal and going over board with portion sizes?" Meaning, when you are making food choices for lunch, have you been filling your plate with mashed potatoes, pasta, bread, biscuits and breaded chicken and breaded steak (the batter for the meat and chicken and all else belong to carbs in List B and portion sizes have gone way beyond that average quarter size round plate. Consequently this will contribute to weight gain. Review the "Meal Blueprint" for more balanced food choices and portion sizes.

Periodically run this checklist and see if you have fallen back to your old habits and make corrections to your actions accordingly and you will see that you will get back on track and will start losing again. **Sometimes it seems that no matter what you do, you stop losing and you hit a plateau. The solution is in the next paragraph.**

"I Hit a Plateau and Stopped Losing Weight after I Have Been Doing Well—What Should I Do?"

After you have lost a good chunk of weight, you might hit a plateau; it seems, no matter what you do, you no longer see pounds coming off. This is normal; we all go through it. After a certain period of time of doing the same activity day in and day out, your brain adapts to that level of activity and prevents further weight loss, but you will still get all the health and disease prevention benefits, and you are able to maintain that loss with your current lifestyle; but further losses become more difficult.

You can remedy this by adding **variety** to the activities you are doing. Doing something different than you are used may stimulate further results. If you have been walking at the same pace and the same distance day in and day out, it's a good idea to use a stationary bicycle next time or an outdoor bicycle as a variety. or if you have access to a gym, then use the elliptical machine for a change. Also, a powerful form of activity that is sure to break that gridlock is to use the "Interval Cycles" as discussed in the activity sections (refer to that action for details).

Also, review the previous section above for additional tips on boosting your weight loss efforts. Having said that, there will come a point after you have mastered making favorable lifestyle choices and lost most of the weight desired, your weight will settle naturally to a comfortable limit. Your goal would be then to maintain and continue making favorable lifestyle choices but not with the goal of losing more weight but to enjoy life and your current energy levels and to celebrate a vibrant life void of lifestyle related diseases or disease complications.

Lifestyle Choices

> **WHAT YOU ABSOLUTELY MUST KNOW AT A GLANCE FROM ACTION STEP 4**
>
> 1. Establish a solid foundation of learning how to build new and favorable habits (as discussed starting on Page 129), and apply these same principles on making favorable food and activity choices, as if you are learning new tasks at a new job. When you make a not-so-good choice, forgive yourself and make a better one next time, just like the initial learning phase at that new job for the first 3-4 weeks, after which you develop a habit of making favorable food and activity choices most of the time.
>
> 2. "Make a Habit" of making favorable food choices and **portion-sizes** (as discussed in "The Meal Structure Blueprint" (starting Page 181). Make food choices more frequently from the entire List A food categories that are beneficial for your health, that prevent disease, and that help you lose weight. Make food choices less frequently from List B.
>
> 3. "Make a Habit" of increasing your level of activity daily as discussed in the "Activity" section (starting on Page 206).
>
> 4. Simple and easy tips that will help you lose weight and boost further weight loss without dieting as discussed in "Simple Tips for Immediate weight loss"(on Page 231). You will lose weight and keep it off because you are not depriving yourself from any food group, but you are making balanced choices. Most importantly, you are able to keep your diabetes under control, prevent all sorts of complications, improve your quality of life and maintain peace of mind.

Action Step 5:
Stress Relief and Management

Your health needs to be good in order for everything else to be good. By taking care of yourself first, you are able to provide care to and for others. If your health is not in good shape, and you are constantly physically and emotionally drained, then your ability to give care to others will be compromised. Consequently, enjoyment of life is nowhere to be found. If you have taken a plane flight, you'll remember that before the plane took off, the flight crew gave the travelers flight instructions. When they got to the part about the oxygen masks that drop if the cabin pressure is down, did they say put the oxygen mask on your child or on yourself first? Of course, you put the oxygen mask on yourself first. Why? If you suffocate, you cannot help others. Likewise, in everyday life, as soon as you start making better lifestyle choices and try to reduce or manage your stress levels, you will be breathing that oxygen first.

Dare to love and reward yourself and accept yourself just the way you are. At this moment, make a lifelong commitment to get into the habit of making better lifestyle choices, and do what it takes to improve your health and reduce your daily stress. It will be good for you and you will see that as you do so inner happiness will start to trickle down your way. I know that every one is capable of doing so.

Stress is a major contributor and a major magnet to potentially harmful conditions such as:

- Weight gain
- Fat accumulation in the abdominal area
- Heart disease
- High blood pressure
- High blood cholesterol
- Diabetes
- Ulcers
- Anxiety disorders
- Depression
- Sleep disturbances
- Daytime fatigue
- Sexual dysfunction in both men and women
- Stress negatively affects relationships, job performance, and worsens any pre-existing health condition such as the ones mentioned above

Studies Have Shown that Only 6% of All Stress We Face Each Day Is Legitimate Stress. The Remaining 94% of all other worries and stresses that plague our lives are anticipated but do not actually happen. This means that the vast majority of the time, we worry too much about a problem that will never happen. That's a terrible waste. Instead of worrying, we should do what we can to prevent the dreaded situations. We need to realize that there are many situations not under our control, and no amount of worrying will affect the outcome. So, RELAX.

Some Real Worries and How People Generally Deal with Them

Some of the real worries and stresses that do fall into the 6% bracket can be any of the following:

- Death of a loved one
- Divorce or abusive relationship
- Debt
- Legal matters
- Illness of self or loved one

These factors do impact our lives in a serious and negative manner, often generating a feeling of impending doom. **Although some of these situations are imposed on us without our consent, we can choose how to deal with them.**

When facing one of these crises, you have a choice of responses. You can take a destructive course of action that will negatively impact your physical and mental well being further, which will weaken you further and not help you face that major challenge that is still in progress. Alternatively, you could deal with that major stress in a positive manner, maintaining your good health and preparing all your body's senses, mentally and physically, and keeping them in good shape to face that challenge head-on and get beyond that obstacle.

It seems to be the course of least resistance for people going through difficult situations to choose behaviors that will compromise their health. Some of the unfavorable and self-destructive ways that many people choose to deal with major stresses are:

- Overeating and, consequently, gaining weight while losing self-esteem, bringing on unwanted diseases or worsening current chronic conditions such as diabetes and high blood pressure.

- Doing nothing or remaining inactive, sedentary, staying home and watching TV and worrying which tend to also bring your way unwanted and uninvited diseases and worsening current ones.
- If the person is a smoker, he/she increases the amount of cigarettes they smoke per day; or ex-smokers return to that old habit, and by doing so, put themselves in harm's way again, thus compounding several fold the risk of various deadly diseases (definitely unwanted at this stressful period you are going through).
- Overusing alcohol and drugs.
- Withdrawing from friends.
- Hurting oneself overtly.
- A combination of many or all of the above.

These choices are not solutions; on the contrary, these choices actually fuel the problems you are experiencing and prevent a speedy recovery from that day's major stress.

You actually have the power within you to choose to deal with that stress in a manner that is favorable for your health. If you find yourself in a negative cycle of self-loathing and self-destruction as a result of major problems, you can turn things around for yourself by **taking charge of your life. You are worth it. No one can pull you out of that situation except yourself. You are capable of taking that first step into a positive territory. Make that decision RIGHT NOW, not later. Seek professional help to find closure for the source of that problem. Without closure, you can't expect to see the light at the end of the tunnel.**

What Are Favorable Ways to Deal with Major Stresses?

1. Dealing with a Bad Relationship or a Troubled Marriage

If you are in a bad relationship, comforting yourself by overeating or smoking will not resolve your problem or remove the source of it. These measures of "comfort" are actually a form of self-punishment, because they hurt only you in the end and do not contribute to helping you deal and overcome the current difficulty you are going through. A solution to the problem is needed, not something to anesthetize you. Seek the type of professional help that can help you find a solution. You might seek a professional or religious counselor to see if the relationship can be improved. A lawyer may be appropriate in the case of a bad marriage that can't be helped through counseling. **If you are in a**

relationship in which you are being abused or your life is in danger, call the police or a crisis line immediately. Inaction is not an option if you are being abused.

2. Dealing with the Loss of a Loved One

If you have lost a loved one, in addition to experiencing grief and loss, you may feel bitter and brokenhearted. I know first hand the sadness that the sudden loss of my precious father has caused my family and me. You will be going through a major mournful phase, and the support of family and friends is paramount during such a difficult time. Don't discount the power of prayer, because prayer, especially in such a time, is a major healer. Seeking religious counseling can be of great support and consolation as well.

Focusing on your own health can be difficult at such times, but you must force yourself to make that choice, hurting yourself by choosing the other unhealthy options discussed above IS NOT THE ANSWER. Neglecting yourself and coping with sorrow by overeating, staying inactive, smoking, or drinking alcohol will do nothing but impact negatively on your health and mental well being. Life is for the living, and we must cherish this miracle of life and participate whole-heartedly in it. By making our health a priority we can prepare ourselves to be well ready to face life's most formidable challenges. So pick up your pieces, start making better food and activity choices as recommended in this guide, decide to quit smoking as soon as possible and my smoking cessation guide "Stop Smoking Today" will offer you a real solution. Seek professional help for your sorrow if you feel that it is not working on your own and keep the support of your friends and family strong. Also start practicing the stress relieving techniques mentioned in the stress-buster section below. Go on, celebrate life, and live the life your passing loved one would want you to live.

3. Dealing with Debt

Being in debt feels like serving a prison sentence, disrupting your life and marriage. Debt can be the mother of all stresses. Seek professional help of a lawyer or an accountant to get out of debt. Your sanity is more important than your credit. You can build your credit back up and learn not to be under the grip of debt and creditors any longer. Live within your means, and if you can't afford something, don't charge it. The burden of seeing your hard-earned money being blown away on interest charges and late fees does not justify that flashy car or that house that you cannot afford. Relieving debt from your shoulders lightens your burden and will bring back your peace of mind. Keep yourself in good health as you face and overcome your challenges, including debt, by making favorable lifestyle choices and using stress-relieving techniques.

4. Legal Matters

If you are currently entangled in a legal matter that is placing tremendous stresses on your life, it is wise to consult a specialized lawyer for advice. Any up front lawyer fees, regardless of how exorbitant they are, will be far cheaper than the tens of thousands of dollars in expenses that will ensue from any legal entanglement later on down the road when things go wrong, and things do go wrong very frequently. Until that matter is resolved, good health and living a stress-free life is paramount to your mental and physical well being and your capacity to fight back and win that legal matter. Choosing appropriate foods and activities and practicing stress-relieving techniques will sharpen your mental quality.

5. Sickness

When you are ill, ask your doctor what exercises would be advisable and what limitations. Work within your limitations, being cautious not to overdo. For instance, if you have severe knee arthritis or you have any kind of leg pain due to diabetes, you will not be able to walk 30 or 45 minutes at once. Instead, walk for ten-minute bouts, three times a day, several times a week. Whenever pain sets in as you are walking, that should be your sign to stop. Pushing beyond your personal limit will make you feel worse. However, by remaining active within your limitations, eating healthy foods, and practicing stress relieving techniques, will help you better cope with other health problems.

One of the most important factors in recovery is attitude. Since illness can cause major stress, pain, and depression, seeking professional counseling could help make a significant difference in your condition.

Major Stress Busters that You Can Start Practicing Right Now:

- Lose weight by making favorable food and activity choices.
- Schedule 30-45 minutes of physical activity 3-5 times a week (Yes! Activity is major stress buster).

- Take a 5 or 10-minute power-walk whenever you are under a stressful situation.

- Maintain a good and balanced sex life, no less frequent than at least 2-4 times a week (research has shown that married couples who have frequent sexual encounters lead less stressful lives and consequently have a better life-expectancy rate than single people who are less sexually active).

- Take ten semi-deep breaths when experiencing stress (if you take deep breath you might feel a little light headed.) When extra oxygen reaches the brain, it relieves stress and promotes a sense of relaxation).

- Practice the following brief powerful relaxation technique that provides immediate relaxation anywhere you are, whether at home or work: shut your eyes for only 2-3 minutes, breathe normally and focus only on your breathing. As you exhale, let your mind focus on the word "relax." If other thoughts start clouding your mind, clear them right away and refocus on your breathing; you can do this several times a day.

- Reward yourself frequently by engaging in activities which bring you personal satisfaction, pleasure or a feeling of well-being such as getting a massage, manicure, pedicure or any other activity that brings you personal satisfaction and pleasure.

- Forgive others and do not hold grudges, and consider praying for those who bring you misery, which will bring you relief.

- Do not expect perfection of yourself, because doing so invariably brings feelings of failure and raises your stress levels.

- Frequently break the monotony of your daily routine by doing something different and fun, for instance, bungee jumping.

- Attend a play, a musical, or a concert with a friend, your spouse or by yourself.

- Allow your home to be your safe haven, leaving all unpleasant thoughts from work or other sources out the door. (If a stressful incident comes to mind, switch your thought immediately to something pleasant and occupy yourself with something other than work such as cutting up some vegetables, cooking, while listening to some relaxing music in the background.

- Think of what brings you peace, balance and happiness; and be sure to live in the moment, not anticipating possible future problems that may not even surface.

- Meet with friends for coffee or activity once or twice a week or more.

- Learn something new or pursue a new hobby, such as gardening, cooking classes, or others of your choice.

- Relax in the evening by dimming the lights, putting on relaxing music, or taking a bubble bath, or watching your favorite TV show.

- Practice aromatherapy by using incense, candles or scented oils. (Be careful of allergies you might have to any scent.)

- Rent a favorite movie and turn your ringers, phones and computer off and allow the movie to take you on a short excursion that evening.

- Do some volunteer work and help others; Sometimes when you put your energy in assisting others, this will make your mind shift focus from your own stresses and bring you some stress relief.

- Organize your house, especially clothes and closets; discarding clothes that you have not worn in two years. Activity will help you forget your problems for a while, and it will create a less cluttered environment which will also reduce stress.

- Buy some new clothes, remembering to stay within your means.

- Change your hairstyle or color.

- Invite friends over for dinner and cook for them.

- Make a fun list of things you would enjoy doing and refer to the list whenever you're stressed or bored.

- Practice relaxation techniques such as meditation and yoga; (see the Meditation Techniques section which follows).

BASIC MEDITATION TECHNIQUE

Lie down on your back, close your eyes, then relax each body muscle within each muscle group, starting with your toes and working your way up to your eyebrows until every muscle is relaxed. Then start breathing more deeply and focus only on your breathing while inhaling and exhaling. Clear out all other thoughts from your mind and as you are breathing out say calming words to yourself such as "relax" with each exhalation. If your mind drifts to various mundane or stressful thoughts, clear these thoughts by refocusing on your breathing. This will have a calming effect on you. You can be creative while focusing on your breathing; imagine an ideal place or sanctuary that brings you peace, such as a favorite vacation spot. The more you practice meditating, the more vivid those pictures of your sanctuary havens will become, and the more you will be in control of your thoughts. You can begin with 5-10 minute per day, and you can progress if you wish, by perhaps taking weekly or multi-weekly yoga classes.

Engage in activities that will benefit your mind, your body, and your health. Take one small step forward at a time, all the while, moving into a positive territory; **climb to the top of the success ladder, whatever that success you'd like to achieve, one step forward at a time. You are worth it, you can do it, and you will succeed.**

> ### What You Absolutely Must Know at a Glance From Action Step 5
>
> - Practicing to manage stress is the final link in regaining control over your diabetes and health.
> - Only 6% of all your worries actually occur and are worth worrying about; don't anticipate what might possibly go wrong, as it often never does and many people waste their time and necessary energy worrying about things that never occur (Page 238).
> - Incorporating stress-relieving techniques in your everyday lifestyle will help you, enormously, in reducing your stress level, managing and bringing your disease under control and consequently improving your quality of life (Page 241).

A Word about Alcohol

Alcohol is a weapon with two sharp edges. Several clinical studies have well established that consuming one drink per day has favorable effects on the heart and may reduce the incidence of heart problems. Those same studies have also shown that when people exceed 2 drinks per day, this same beneficial substance turns into a deadly weapon. **One drink constitutes one beer or one glass of wine or one ounce of hard liquor or spirits.**

Here Are Some Benefits of Balanced Alcohol Consumption:
- Alcohol dilates the blood vessels and contributes to keeping them elastic and flexible, thus reducing incidents of heart disease.
- Alcohol reduces blood pressure mildly.
- Red wine contains powerful antioxidants called tannins that may prevent heart disease.
- Alcohol reduces stress levels if only 1-2 drinks are consumed every day or every other day, if desired.
- Alcohol mildly increases the good cholesterol levels (HDL).

During my pharmacy practice, I was amazed and still am amazed as to the ways in which people often misinterpret various information. One time I was counseling a patient, and when I asked him about alcohol consumption, he said, "Oh well, you know, I know that alcohol is good for ya, so I might have a couple of drinks a day." His wife immediately interjected and said, "Well, let's make that more like 3 or 4 drinks of tall whiskey glasses per day."

I felt she was trying to reach out to me so I can help sway her husband against drinking that much. So I proceeded to provide the recommended guidelines about alcohol and suggested he drop back his drinking to an ounce of whiskey every day or every other day instead of the number of drinks he was currently imbibing. I also explained that exceeding these limits would quickly jeopardize his health and put him in grave danger. I was not sure whether my recommendation had fallen on deaf ears, but I did what I had to do; it's up to him to act on the information he was given.

The Severe Consequences of Consuming More than Two Alcoholic Drinks Per Day:

- Liver damage
- Cancer of the liver and the colon
- Ulcers
- Addiction/alcoholism
- Sexual dysfunction in men and women
- Erective dysfunction
- **Weight gain**
- Worsens diabetes control
- Worsening of blood pressure
- Worsening of heart disease
- Insomnia and trouble sleeping
- Worsens or causes depression and anxiety
- Interacts with medications such as antidepressants, anti-anxiety, anti-psychotics, narcotic pain killers, and most medications that are metabolized by the liver

Consuming Alcohol and Diabetes

People who have diabetes can also receive the same benefits of moderate alcohol consumption; about 1-2 drinks every day or every other day, as mentioned earlier. If you don't currently consume alcohol, you don't have to start now in order to gain health benefits. You can gain health benefits by making favorable food and activity choices. However, when you exceed the amounts previously mentioned, alcohol will most definitely and negatively impact your diabetes control. If you are diabetic and choose to consume alcohol, make sure to do so within the recommended guidelines of 1-2 drinks every day or every other day or less frequently.

Advice to College Students and All Those Who Consume Large Amounts of Alcohol

Anytime you guzzle large amounts of alcohol in any one evening, even if it's once a weekend or once a month, you are causing damage to your liver that could be irreversible. College students think they are still young and invincible, and that health problems happen to others. You can be young, alcoholic, and prone to all the ailments listed previously in this section if you consume more than 2 drinks per day, consistently. The college student drinkers of today can become the alcoholics, smokers, drug addicts and cancer patients of tomorrow in as little as 5-10 years down the road. Don't become one of them. **Moderation can be adopted at any age.**

Who Should Not Consume Any Alcohol:

- If you are currently diagnosed with any kind of liver problems or if your doctor suspects any liver problems.
- If your doctor advises you not to consume alcohol for any specific condition.
- If you have been an alcoholic in the past.
- If you have any other substance addiction.
- If you are taking any medications belonging to the class of drug listed in the section above that is entitled "The Severe Consequences of Consuming More Than Two Drinks Per Day."

Women and Men: Boost Your Sexual Health at Any Age

Sexual desires or libido for both men and women have decreased in the last two decades, coinciding with an all-time record number of obese and overweight people. Poor lifestyle choices are largely to be blamed for this surging obesity epidemic and the resulting sexual dysfunction it has caused men and women.

In reality, as mentioned before that an estimated whopping 60% of the American population is overweight or obese. Clinical studies show that the majority of these suffer from at least one kind of sexual dysfunction. It is estimated that over **40% of women suffer from sexual dysfunction**, such as low sexual desires (libido), problems with arousal, and pain during intercourse. For the male counterpart, **about 30 million men in the United States suffer from erectile dysfunction**, premature ejaculation, and loss of sexual desires. Between 60-70% of males over 65 develop these problems. The American Foundation for Urologic Disease estimates that only 5-10% of these men seek professional help. **The good news is that there is a solution for any sexual challenge for men and women at any age.**

The Arousal Process and the Problems that Could Affect It

Arousal, in both men and women, involves a sequence of events, starting with seeing, hearing or touching (any of these stimuli or any combination of them are part of the arousal process). These stimuli are transmitted to the brain through nerve impulses. In turn, the brain sends these impulses to the spinal cord and, consequently, to all the erogenous areas of the body in particular, to the genital areas. Blood flow through blood vessels begins to engorge the genital areas in preparation for physical arousal of the genitals and heightened sensitivity in those areas. At this stage, the vagina in women becomes engorged with blood and causes the arousal of the vaginal organ; and in the male, blood rushes into the two chambers that run the length of the penis. Responses in structures such as muscle, fibrous tissue, and blood vessels cause the erection. Sexual dysfunction can happen if any of these systems are affected by physiological and/or psychological problems.

The Main Factors Causing Sexual Dysfunction in Men and Women

Sexual dysfunction is the result of factors that we have control over and, therefore, can change. Poor lifestyle choices are largely to blame for the sexual dysfunction in men as well as women. Unhealthy eating habits, smoking and inactivity are largely to blame, not only for the obesity epidemic, but also for causing diseases which lead to sexual dysfunction in men and women. Obesity reduces sexual function by contributing to poor health and a poor psychological state, possibly creating fear of sexual failures, low self-esteem, depression, stress, and anxiety. Obesity and smoking cause major preventable diseases such as diabetes, high blood pressure, high cholesterol, kidney dysfunction and heart disease. Sexual dysfunction can result from any of these physical conditions and is compounded by the combination of psychological problems.

All of these diseases affect various aspects of the sexual arousal process in both men and women if there is damage to the nerves, blood vessels and smooth muscles inside these blood vessels. In men, these events cause dysfunction of the fibrous tissue and blood flow in the penis, thus disrupting almost every aspect of the sexual arousal process.

Additional Causes of Sexual Dysfunction Are:

- Limited range of motion in people who are overweight or obese due to excess fat that gets in the way of the genital areas leading to limited sexual positions.
- Substance abuse: alcohol, cigarettes, street drugs.
- Liver problems.
- Prostate surgery for men and endometriosis and/or removal of the ovaries or uterus for women.
- Cancers in men such as prostate and testicular cancer; cancers in women such as cancers of the uterus, breast, or ovaries.

Common Medications that Cause Sexual Dysfunction:

- Some blood pressure medications such as beta blockers.
- Antidepressants (excluding Wellbutrin).
- Sedatives (such as Valium, Xanax or Klonopin).
- Appetite suppressants (such as amphetamines, Adipex, Ionamin, any Phentermine products, and Meridia).
- Prolonged use (weeks and months) of antihistamines.

- Anti-psychotics (such as Haldol, Zyprexa, Seroquel, and Risperdal).
- Chronic usage of narcotic pain killers (Morphine, Oxycodone, Hydrocodone-related-products and codeine-related-products).
- Nitroglycerin (oral pills and patches used for heart disease).
- Some diuretics such as Hydrochlorothiazide.
- Prostate cancer treatment, which includes female hormones such as Lupron.
- Illegal-drug-usage (such as Heroin, Cocaine, LSD, Amphetamines and Methamphetamines).
- Hormonal insufficiencies:

  In Women: menopause causes a reduction in both the female hormones and testosterone (the male hormone which is produced in small amounts in women's' bodies and which is responsible in part for the sexual arousal phase).

  In Men: Andropause, the reduction in the levels of testosterone, affects the arousal phase in men.
- Men experiencing erection problems due to obesity, diabetes, or high blood pressure or high cholesterol can also experience psychological challenges, such as: depression, anxiety and fear of sexual failure, causing reluctance to attempt sexual approaches.

I was on duty once when a middle-aged man discreetly approached the pharmacy consultation window wanting help. He told me he was a two-year prostate cancer survivor and had undergone radiation and female hormone treatment. He told me his cancer went away, but so did his sexual life. He had trouble "getting it up" and shared with me his lack of confidence in approaching women for fear of sexual failure.

Not being the man he used to be was a tremendous blow to his self-esteem and ego. At times, he wished he were not alive so he wouldn't have to go through this humiliation and disruption in his life. He asked if there were any over-the-counter medications he could use to help his condition. Another concern of his was that he was without insurance.

I could really sense his tremendous anxiety and suffering. Erectile dysfunction is devastating to most men. I empathized with his emotional situation, assuring him that millions like him are suffering from this problem, and that there is help available. Probing further about his general health condition, the medication he was taking and his current lifestyle, I realized he was leading a sedentary life, eating lots of fried food and was overweight. He was also taking a beta-blocker for blood pressure.

I gave him suggestions for increasing his daily activity and making more balanced food choices. The resultant loss of weight could be a tremendous boost for his sexual health. I advised him to seek the help of a doctor for treatment, regardless of how much the doctor's visit cost, since this investment would help him claim his sexual life back. I also indicated to him the availability of several reliable and proven oral medications for sexual dysfunction, along with several other options in case the pills did not work. A couple of months later, he came back to tell me about the improvement in his sexual life after losing about 7 or 8 pounds of weight, becoming more active, and taking a pill prescribed by his doctor.

The Benefits of a Healthy Sexual Life

The benefits of a healthy sexual life are enormous to the well being of our minds, bodies, and our social life. A sexual frequency of about 3-5 times a week provides benefits such as:

- Increase in self-esteem
- Stress reduction and relaxation
- Decreased incidence of heart disease
- Decreased blood pressure
- Weight loss and weight management
- Increase in work productivity
- Better life expectancy.

The energy demands required from almost all of our body muscles, such as arms, chest, shoulders, legs, buttocks, back, and abdominal muscles during sexual encounters help us lose weight by burning more calories than if we were not actively engaged in sex.

Libido Booster for Men and Women in Three Easy Steps

Jumpstart your sexual life now by doing 3 things:

1. Lose weight by making favorable lifestyle choices such as becoming more active, making balanced food selections and quitting smoking. As you take these steps, your heart, arteries and blood vessels will begin healing. Regaining good health and becoming more physically fit, along with the healing of your vital organs are absolute prerequisites to boosting your sex life.

2. Seek the help of your doctor. There will most likely be a treatment solution to whatever sexual dysfunction you might have.

3. Keep your diabetes, cholesterol, blood pressure, and heart disease under control by keeping your sugar, blood pressure, and cholesterol levels within recommended ranges as discussed in Action Step 3; this will boost the sexual arousal process in men and women.

Women

WHAT TREATMENTS ARE AVAILABLE FOR SEXUAL DYSFUNCTION IN WOMEN?

Hormone Replacement

Women experiencing female hormone shortage as a result of menopause or surgically induced menopausal conditions may experience diminished sexual desires, painful sex due to vaginal dryness, flushing, bone loss, and increased risk of heart disease. These factors can be effectively addressed with the use of hormone replacement therapy (HRT) for a limited period of time between 2-5 years. HRT can be administered orally, through gels or creams applied topically to the vagina or other areas of the body, or administered inside the vagina (each product is available in a different form and has various usage sites and your doctor will choose the one appropriate for you).

NOTE: In the past few years, **several studies revealed that women taking hormone replacement therapy for over five years are at risk of developing heart disease, blood clots, breast cancer, and uterine cancer,** especially when combined with other unfavorable lifestyle risk factors, such as smoking, obesity, and sedentary lifestyles. Prolonged usage of HRT is no longer the practice, and there are now effective drugs other than hormones that are available to treat various conditions, such as osteoporosis and high cholesterol but which do not put women at risk.

Females who have been taking oral hormones for more than 2-3 years should discuss the various options available to them with their doctor. Each situation needs to be considered individually. In some instances, prolonged use of HRT may be warranted and together you and your doctor can make that decision.

In other situations, the doctor may elect to prescribe local vaginal creams or gels to effectively relieve sexual issues. Local use of vaginal hormone creams releases negligible amounts of the hormones to the rest of your body through the blood while locally and effectively relieving menopausal symptoms such as flushing, enhancing sexual desires/

libido, improving arousal and inducing natural vaginal lubrication, and relieving painful sex. Women who currently have or have had cancer are generally discouraged from using hormone creams; however, there are lubricants on the market, which will relieve vaginal dryness. Using warmth-producing vaginal lubricants helps resolve vaginal dryness issues and promote a heightened level of arousal.

Part of the sexual challenge after menopause is not only the lack of female hormones, but also the lack of the male hormone, testosterone, which is secreted in a woman's body in small amounts. It is testosterone that is mostly responsible for inducing sexual desires or libido in women. At menopause, testosterone is no longer produced, resulting in diminished libido. Discuss treatment options with your doctor.

Estratest

The Estratest drug that is available in two strengths combines estrogen and testosterone. Taking one of these hormone pills daily may help increase a woman's libido. The doctor will address individualized treatment approaches for each woman in terms of her medical profile and reaction to drugs. Changes in the treatment plan may result on the basis of effectiveness.

Viagra

Viagra for women? Currently Viagra is only indicated for men with Erectile Dyscfunction.

However, some doctors have been prescribing it for women and with satisfying results. I happened to fill Viagra prescriptions for a couple women. Upon counseling, each of those women (one was about 72 years young) claimed that they were getting the results they were looking for and that "Viagra has been working just fine." See the discussion about Viagra in the men's section further down.

Over-the-Counter Vaginal Lubricants

Using over-the-counter vaginal lubricants and warming gels relieves painful intercourse, and the warming effect caused by these formulas dilates the blood vessels and draws more blood to the vaginal area, consequently heightening sensations and improving arousal.

DHEA

DHEA was shown in one study to effectively raise the levels of male hormones and consequently increase sexual desires or libido in women. Check with your doctor prior to starting DHEA treatment.

Over-the-Counter Herbal Hormone-Like Products

Black Cohosh, an active ingredient in many over-the-counter products and is used to treat the symptoms of natural and surgically induced menopause, such as hot flashes and sweating. The use of over-the-counter Black Cohosh products is not intended to replace hormone therapy, nor is it to be used for prolonged periods of time. It can be used intermittently for 3-6 months at a time. Black Cohosh can help Women relieve menopausal symptoms, such as flushing, vaginal dryness, and sweating and may improve their sexual drive.

Post-Menopausal Symptom Relief without the Use of Medicinals

Some factors may worsen the symptoms of menopause and consequently the sexual mood, such as consuming spicy food, being in hot and humid environments, sedentary lifestyles, lack of cool hydration, and being overweight. By avoiding these situations and by making better lifestyle choices and, when needed, by using Black Cohosh products for short periods of time may help.

Pregnancy, Birth Control, Vaginal Infections and Women Who Have Diabetes

Women of childbearing age being treated for diabetes need to be using effective birth control if they are not intending to become pregnant, since many of the oral diabetes medications are contraindicated during pregnancy. There are several and highly effective **Oral Contraceptive** choices that your doctor can appropriately prescribe for you. Barrier methods such as Diaphragms and IUDs (Intra Uterine Device) can be reliable forms of contraception but due to your body weight changes and their chance of raising the incidence of vaginal bacterial and yeast infections in women with diabetes makes them fall behind the oral contraceptives.

Diabetic women who don't have their sugar under control have already an increased frequency of vaginal infections interfering with their sexual activity rendering the barrier method of contraception not ideal. Solution; bring your sugar under control as described in all of the Action Steps. For fungal yeast infections you can use the Over-The-Counter vaginal creams or suppositories such as Monistat, Gyne-Lotrimin, Mycelex or the store brand equivalent of these products (the 1,3 or 7 days are equally effective). For unhealed or recurrent yeast infections your doctor may elect to put you on oral Diflucan treatment (by prescription only). For vaginal bacterial infections your doctor may prescribe prescription vaginal creams. The quicker you bring your sugar under control the quicker you heal and have fewer vaginal infections; the faster you can go back to an uninterrupted, healthy and fulfilling sexual frequency.

Diabetic women of child bearing age who choose to become pregnant and start a family should have no problem doing so and can expect to have a healthy pregnancy and baby provided that they have no other reproductive disorders or challenges. However, as we discussed in Gestational diabetes (see Action Step 1), blood sugar needs to be brought under control (below 95mg/dl on a fasting state and below 120 mg/dl 2 hours after a meal) in order to avoid harm to the baby. The treating physician will most likely switch women with Type 2 diabetes on oral medications to Insulin during pregnancy. Insulin is safe for use during pregnancy.

Sexual Dysfunction Caused by Medications

A complete list of the classes of medication that can cause sexual dysfunction is found earlier in this chapter. If suffering from sexual dysfunction while on any medication belonging to the following classes, you should contact a doctor and let him or her know of this problem so medications can be changed. We will discuss two of the most widely used category of drugs, which might cause sexual dysfunction: antidepressants and antihistamines.

Antidepressants

Women experience higher rates of depression than men. Medications for depression belonging to the "SSRI" (Selective Serotonin Reuptake Inhibitors) group such as Prozac, Zoloft, Paxil, are most notorious for causing anorgasmia, meaning lack of orgasm. Changing the medications to a different class of antidepressant may alleviate this condition. Wellbutrin is an effective drug used to treat depression and may have a unique effect of actually increasing sexual desire in both genders and could promote a slight weight loss. One woman, after she had been put on Wellbutrin, was reported having a spontaneous orgasm while shopping. Prior to Wellbutrin, she was experiencing sexual challenges. However, all drugs have possible side effects. Wellbutrin may raise the chance of having seizures for people who are predisposed to that condition.

Depression and consequent sexual dysfunction can be alleviated through maintaining a healthy weight range and remaining active. One woman I know took up square dancing and found that remaining active provided an effective antidote for depression and tremendously improved her mood. Her sexual function improved in the process. It is difficult to dance with friendly and lively people and be depressed at the same time.

Antihistamines

Antihistamines such as Claritin, Allegra, and Zyrtec, when taken on a regular basis for weeks and months cause vaginal dryness and consequently painful intercourse. This will cause women taking these antihistamines to be less likely to engage in sexual activity; consequently, their sexual health is compromised. Women on antihistamines experiencing any kind of sexual dysfunction and vaginal dryness should consult their doctor about alternative treatments for allergies and are good candidates for warmth-producing vaginal lubricants.

Future Drugs to Treat Sexual Dysfunction in Women

Alista (this drug is not yet on the market): Alista is a product containing the active ingredient Alprostadil, which is currently being developed for topical vaginal use by women. Alprostadil is currently used to treat sexual dysfunction in men. Alprostadil, when applied as a cream to the vaginal and clitoral areas, causes dilation of blood vessels and produces blood engorgement and significant increases in sexual arousal.

Men

WHAT TREATMENTS ARE AVAILABLE FOR SEXUAL DYSFUNCTION IN MEN?

Improving lifestyle choices, losing weight by making better food and activity choices as discussed throughout this guide, and avoiding medication that causes sexual dysfunction, all help to eliminate Erectile Dysfunction and help men at any age return to sexual activity. **Low blood thyroid and testosterone** levels contribute to Erectile Dysfunction; your doctor will check your blood levels of these 2 substances and prescribe appropriate treatments to rectify those deficiencies. Up to 50% of all men who have diabetes have some form of sexual dysfunction. Advances in medical interventions catapulted the choices available to treat Erectile Dysfunction to an all-time high and revolutionized men's sexual health.

Although psychological support is important, however, treatment of erectile problems by taking medications orally has become prevalent, starting with Viagra, which became available in 1998. Let's see what is currently available and what the differences between medications are: Viagra arrived first in 1998, and then came Levitra and then Cialis.

	Comparison of Medications For Erectile Problems
Viagra	<ul><li>(Available in 25, 50, and 100 mgs.)</li><li>Time to erection: 1 hour</li><li>Duration of activity: up to 5 hours</li></ul>
Levitra	<ul><li>(Available in 10 and 20 mgs.)</li><li>Time to erection: 15 minutes</li><li>Duration of activity: up to 5 hours</li></ul>
Cialis	<ul><li>(Available in 5, 10, and 20 mgs.)</li><li>Time to erection: 15-30 minutes</li><li>Duration of activity: up to 36 hours</li></ul>

All these medications are good choices and are equally effective in producing erections, but there are advantages to the newer agents. For instance, Levitra and Cialis can produce an erection within only 15 minutes, which brings back spontaneity to sexual relations. Cialis' effect can last up to 36 hours and longer, making it the best choice for spontaneity. A man can take one Cialis tablet just 3 times a week and can initiate sex and get an erection anytime. With that advantage, Cialis has brought back normal sexual lives and spontaneity to couples.

To clarify, duration of activity means that, at any time during those 36 hours, sex can be initiated and an erection is highly likely to happen; the erection will not last for that entire 5 or 36 hours, depending on which drug is used. In fact, an erection lasting more than 3 or 4 hours constitutes an emergency and needs to be dealt with immediately, as discussed in the upcoming section.

Common Side Effects

Side effects of these drugs are generally mild and transient. Some common side effects are: facial flushing, headache, upset stomach, back pain or pain in the muscles.

A Rare but Potential Side Effect

Any drug taken orally or used topically to treat sexual dysfunction may cause a rare but potential side effect called *Priapism* or prolonged erection. Any time you have a prolonged erection lasting more than a 3 or 4 hours, seek immediate emergency help.

Who Should Not Take Viagra, Levitra, or Cialis:

- Men who had heart attacks or strokes in the last 6 months or who have unstable blood pressure or heart disease.
- Men taking drugs that will further drop their blood pressure or dilate their blood vessels such as nitroglycerin taken by mouth, under the tongue, or in a patch form (blood pressure may drop considerably causing light headedness and fainting).
- Men taking drugs belonging to the Alpha Blocker class such as: Clonidine, Prazosin, Doxazosin, or Terazosin, with the exception of Flomax. Flomax can be used instead. Cutting the dosage of these Alpha Blockers in half may be an option to alleviate drug interaction (blood pressure may drop considerably causing light headedness and fainting).
- Men who consume more than an occasional alcoholic drink (blood pressure may drop considerably causing light headedness and fainting).

A Word of Caution

When taking Viagra, Levitra, or Cialis, especially while also taking other blood pressure-lowering medication, and/or drinking alcohol, one should avoid standing quickly from a seated or lying position or from a bending position where one's head falls below the horizontal plane. Each of these drugs mentioned above cause your blood vessels to dilate. When these drugs are combined, the dilation may become excessive.

Standing abruptly could cause a sudden drop in blood pressure and create a possible occurrence of light-headedness or passing out, a hazardous as well as embarrassing situation. Consequently, aerial sexual maneuvering and acrobatics are discouraged, as well as standing up quickly to perform a standing sexual position. A way of avoiding a sudden drop in blood pressure is to sit on the edge of the bed for a few seconds and then stand slowly.

OTHER AVAILABLE TREATMENTS OR DEVICES FOR SEXUAL DYSFUNCTION

Older products have been used but with various degrees of success, and although they have fallen out of favor, they are still a viable option to treat Erectile Dysfunction.

Muse

A rice-like suppository, Alprostadil, is loaded in a pre-filled syringe and inserted from the tip of the penis halfway down. It causes local increases in blood flow, and an erection will ensue within five or ten minutes, lasting thirty to sixty minutes. Shortcomings include that this procedure is only 40% effective, does not allow for spontaneity, and has a shorter window of action than pills.

Testosterone Treatment

If your doctor finds out from running blood tests that your testosterone levels are low then he or she may elect to put you on testosterone treatment to help with resolving your Erectile Dysfunction condition. Low blood levels of testosterone can reduce sexual desires (Libido) in men and contribute to Erectile Dysfunction. In that case, your doctor may prescribe any of the many testosterone products available such as pills to be taken orally, injections in the muscle, gels to be applied to upper body areas such as upper arm and shoulders or patches to be applied on dry shaven skin covering the testicles or on dry shaven skin in other areas of the body such as the abdomen, upper arms, back, shoulders and thighs depending on each formulation.

Local Injections in the Penis

Drugs causing blood vessel dilation such as Papaverine or Prostaglandin E are injected in the shaft of the penis. They are about 80% effective but not well accepted for apparent reasons. They cause problems such as prolonged erections (Priapism), sudden drop in blood pressure, pain at the site of injection, and local build up of fibrous tissue.

Vacuum Devices

Vacuum devices consist of hollow tubes connected to an outside manual pump. Once the penis is inserted in them the pump is activated to create a vacuum in the process, causing blood to be engorged in the penis thus causing an erection that can last for several minutes. They have been effective for some men but interfere with spontaneity and their use is limited for his purpose.

Surgery

Surgery includes local vascular surgery and placing a prosthesis inside the penis. **There will be no visible trace on the body of the device or the pump**. The pumping site is under the skin and can be activated discretely by placing pressure on the pump under the skin in the scrotum (the testicles sac) area, which causes it to inflate and cause erection when needed. There is a rare risk of infection and failure of the device. Typically the success and satisfaction rate for these implants can be about 95% as claimed by the major implant manufacturers such as American Medical Systems and Mentor. The implant device may be guaranteed for life. **Your insurance may cover this procedure**. Check with your urologist for further details.

Premature Ejaculation

This is a serious burden affecting about 20% of all men; some causes include:

- Poor health
- Inactivity
- Prostate infections
- Diabetes
- Some narcotic pain killers
- Sexual inexperience
- Infrequent sexual intercourse
- Overly heightened arousal
- Lack of understanding of sexual responses
- Poor sexual performance

This problem, although not life-threatening, tremendously affects the quality of life of those men and their sexual partners.

Premature ejaculation has a negative impact on men's sexual health and functioning. It causes sexual anxiety, fear of trying, decrease in arousal, decreased satisfaction with intercourse, and fear of not obtaining an erection, which could lead to Erectile Dysfunction. The man in this situation is less likely to discuss the matter with his mate or his doctor and may suffer from low self-esteem.

Some Effective Available Solutions for Premature Ejaculation:

- Anesthetics applied topically to the penis have been shown to be about 70-80% effective in prolonging the climb to ejaculation. A word of caution is the overuse of these topical anesthetic may cause a loss of ejaculation for the male user and for the female mate a loss of orgasm due to vaginal numbness
- "SS" cream is a topical herbal cream made from nine herbs and has shown to be about 80- 90% effective when applied to the penis
- Wearing multiple condoms to reduce sensation
- Masturbation before intercourse

Dapoxetine, an oral medication that is being reviewed by the FDA for approval, has been shown to provide promising results; once it is on the market it can be used on an as-needed basis.

Any medical intervention to any sexual dysfunction will not be complete or fully successful unless the other non-pharmacological factors of the interactions among the sexes are addressed. After many readings on the intriguing topic of a healthy sexuality, here is my contribution on this topic.

ADD A SPARK AND BOOST YOUR SEXUAL LIFE

Anyone can boost their sexual life with their partner by adopting an open-minded approach, realizing there is always room for improvement, and by becoming more sensitive to their partner's needs. Consequently, this may help you have a more fulfilling sexual life and contribute to improving sexual dysfunction. There are several factors that play an important role in a healthy sexual relationship with your spouse or mate; remember, research confirms, when people:

- Engage in sexual activity at least 2-3 times a week
- Make favorable lifestyle choices
- Keep their weight under control by making balanced food and activity choices
- Quit smoking

They drastically decrease the incidence of heart disease. Here are ways to boost your sexual life now.

COMMUNICATE, LISTEN AND RESPOND TO YOUR PARTNER'S NEEDS

Open communication leads to dialogue both ways, and dialogue and compromise lead to problem-solving. Problem solving leads to conflict resolution as well as stress reduction. When stress and anxiety are reduced, you can have a more fulfilled, healthy and rewarding sexual relationship with your partner. Openly discuss any problem right away, and don't let it build up. Once solved, get it off your shoulders and don't bring up that same issue in future conflicts again, and move on.

POSSIBLE SOLUTIONS FOR RELIEVING SEXUAL ANXIETY AND IMPROVING PERFORMANCE AND AROUSAL

Say your partner asks you to perform a certain act or position with her or him that you are not comfortable doing. Discuss that situation openly with your partner and explain why you prefer not to go through with it, or ask if you could do something different, in lieu of that requested position, which could be equally rewarding. If you keep this problem and others unresolved, then this may cause you sexual performance anxiety, which may lead to Erectile Dysfunction.

Or how about, just for a change, try what she or he has requested from you, maybe in a slightly different version, and just remember that human beings are adaptable. If you repeat something several times, then you may adapt to it and like it. In other words, do what she/he wants for a change and if you don't like it than openly discuss it with your partner and you may offer substitutes.

For instance, if you don't like performing oral sex, then there are some condom or edible lubricants with all sorts of flavors that you can buy from the specialized shops that you can use which will resolve and enhance that situation. or if there are any sexual positions that you are not comfortable in doing, then try to come up with a slightly different version to fulfill your partner's needs. Communicating with your partner, listening and keeping a dialogue going does not make you less of a man or a woman. When you do these things, when you listen to your partner's needs make the effort and try to find compromises and solutions then your life and relationship will be much more rewarding and giving.

Here's another common problem that happens in couples' bedrooms. Say you're in bed and about to initiate sexual contact with your spouse or mate and your spouse brings up the financial challenges that are facing you or that drastic legal matter that you are facing. These are serious topics and can bring tremendous anxiety and can be a major sexual turnoff to any healthy relationship and can impede sexual arousal.

There is a time for every situation to be discussed, and definitely discussing these matters in the safe haven of your bedroom is not the time for it. Leave all such serious issues that could bring anxiety to a different time, say during daytime, and definitely not during intimate contact. If you immediately become upset and do not discuss this matter with your spouse and explain openly that these discussions have brought you tremendous anxiety and that this is not the place and time to discuss such a topic, and if you keep it inside, then this builds up sexual anxiety performance, which then again, can lead to sexual arousal challenges to both genders.

Open-ended communications with your spouse, such as telling him or her to postpone the discussion of this topic to a later time, (bring this up before you become upset) can pay off by having you both spare yourselves the anxiety of such conversations and enjoy a fulfilling and a relaxing sexual encounter.

Foreplay and Proper Timing

If your wife does not confront you with the facts that you have not been sensitive to her sexual needs or if you have been married for a while and don't know when the last time your spouse had an orgasm, then you have a growing and unpredictable problem. The desire-killer in the bedroom is when your wife or spouse or partner seems to be withdrawn from the whole sexual act because your performance duration is anywhere between 5-10 minutes, then you roll back and sink into a deep sleep while she is just getting started.

Men, you are in a very bad situation if you have been going through a similar scenario and not communicated with your partner as to whether she was enjoying your sexual encounters or not, or worse, perhaps she has brought up this matter and you have not done anything about it. Building good relationships, including sexual relationships, takes a lot of on-going, open-ended communication with both partners. Relationships start with two-way communication, listening and responding to each other's needs.

Open-ended questions such as, "What can I do better to improve?" or "How can I stimulate you in a more pleasurable way?" or "How can I do something different to get you to enjoy what we're doing?" should always be ongoing during sexual encounters. Men, if you don't realize by now that women have different timing and need a longer time spent on foreplay before they can achieve orgasm, then you must have just dropped from a different planet. Every woman is different. You need to know the timing of your partner. Some women can have an orgasm after 10 minutes of foreplay, and some others may take 30-40 minutes of foreplay before they can achieve orgasm, and in very different ways. When your partner is not getting enough sexually aroused and satisfied then you cannot ultimately either and that can definitely be a source of sexual dysfunction for both of you.

You need to find out what it takes to get your partner to have an orgasm and respond to her needs and desires. Sexual dissatisfaction is one of two major reasons for relationship breakups and divorce. The other reasons are financial challenges. All of the woman's body can be a love-artist's canvas, a trigger-point for sexual desires, and not only the erogenous areas. Spending enough time in foreplay is crucial for your partner's achieving her sexual height.

Every inch of her skin is a turn-on, so kisses, strokes and caresses all over the body in a systemic way or in an unpredictable fashion are all factors that will heighten your partner's sexual response. And men, do not forget oral sex; the majority of men enjoy receiving it, however, only a minority enjoy giving it to their partners.

More than 80% of women can only achieve orgasm through oral sex. If you don't already perform it, consider trying it. Since only a minority of men performs oral sex, then the remaining majority of women are missing a lot of enjoyment. Men, be guided by your partner as to what is the best way to go about it. Try to help her have her orgasm, be a giver sometimes and not always a taker and get communications going to achieve the best outcomes. During her sexual slow down, the attention you give your wife or partner and proper stimulation will be a tremendous aid to any treatment she is using for low sexual desires or Libido. Your active interest in her needs is a boost to her arousal and to improving her sexual desires. The rewards to both your sexual function and health and to your relationship are enormous for your partner and you.

Women, in turn, can return favors; then it's a mutual act of fulfillment. Women, your men, especially those sexually challenged and using treatment for sexual dysfunction, can tremendously benefit from a foreplay period. Likewise, the man's whole body and skin areas are canvases and receptacles for pleasure upon touch or any other form of stimulation. Men may also need a direct stimulation to the penis via oral and/or manual means and requiring more grip pressure to the penis and more time to achieve a full erection. So again, open ended communication and being sensitive to his needs are paramount to a long term fulfilling sexual life and can be an integral aid to his medications in achieving lasting erections and consequently to your sexual satisfaction.

Regardless of how great we think we are in bed, we must be open to change and to constructive criticism. Regardless of how old we get, we can always improve.

Variety

Variety. If you keep trying the same sexual positions in the same room at the same time, then it does not take a rocket scientist to figure out that your sexual life is boring, unfulfilling, and you're missing out on a lot of sparks. Try variety for a change, and keep it fun. Change your routine, dare and try new sexual positions, new unusual places, and new accessories; jump-start your sexual performance now. This will also be a major complement to the medications you are using to improve your sexual function.

Think back to when you first met, when you used to get intimate in all kinds of ways and all kinds of places. Maybe it is time to relive the past and add a twist to it. Take the opportunity when the kids are out, or make attempts to send them out to your in-laws or a trusted party and try re-living your sexual fantasies in places other than the same bedroom. It is essential to periodically take such time out, even if it's for an afternoon or a couple of afternoons a week.

Better yet, send the kids out periodically to friends or in-laws for a whole weekend getaway, then check in at a hotel or a cabin in some faraway place by a mountain or a lake and relive your sexual fantasies.

Remember, you and your partner were there before your kids came along. You and your partner need to breathe oxygen first before you are able to provide it to others and to your kids. Both of you are the most important factor in the relationship. Neglecting each other will not let the family grow and will be counter-productive. So take the time out and spend that quality time with each other, and keep your relationship fresh.

BE A GIVER

The happiest couples are made up of two givers. The least effective couples are comprised of two takers. Learn the power and pleasure of giving. Try it for a change, not only in bed but also in all aspects of your life, and watch your relationship with your spouse take off to new heights.

For instance, next time you're making love with your spouse or mate, try this powerful technique. Give her pleasure and orgasm first. Whatever it takes, stimulate her, with extended foreplay according to her needs, and use oral sex if she enjoys it, until she achieves her orgasm. Keep trying with discussion and comments until you succeed. Your payoff will be worthwhile. This will make you a better lover and eventually will make you a better person, a giver.

RESPECT

Respect is a major performance-enhancer in couples. Your interaction with any other person should be based on respect. The same should apply to your spouse or mate towards you. Respect each other and be sensitive to each other's needs, then watch your marriage bond get stronger, and also watch your sexual performance peak.

RENEW YOUR VOWS

Periodically, renew your vows and strengthen the bond between you, and don't take each other for granted. Each of you as male or female does not have a specific job that you have to do; but you do it because it is an act of love and because you want to do it and not have to do it or it is expected of you. In other words, your wife's job is not to be in the kitchen cooking for you and raising the kids only. Your job is not only to go to work and provide for your family. Both of you are partners in this relationship and with open-ended communication; respect and love that go both ways you will build a strong bond.

Mention frequently that you love each other, and thank each other for everything each of you does for the other; this is a must in every relationship.

ROMANCE AND ROMANTIC ENVIRONMENT

Creating a romantic environment at home can be a major stress buster and a booster to sexual function. Candlelight, scented candles, incense, calm music, dimmed lights, gentle massages, taking bubble baths with lit candles while sipping on a glass of wine or champagne or while having a relaxing gourmet dinner should be frequent occurrences. Keep all bickering, all anxiety-causing topics, and all stresses or work-related issues out of the bedroom. **Your quiet evening time at home with your spouse or partner should be your safe haven and must not be polluted by anticipated stresses**. Give all your attention to your partner and cater to each other's needs.

Respect each other's boundaries and comfort zones; this is crucial to a successful marriage or relationship. It is a must, especially during intimacy, to respect each others' feelings, likes and dislikes, and it is paramount to a healthy and growing sexual relationship with your spouse or partner and a booster to sexual function and a buster to sexual dysfunction.

If you have any type of sexual dysfunction, now you know you are not alone. You should not feel ashamed or stigmatized by any health concern you might have, including any sexual challenges. You are only human, and humans experience all types of health-related issues throughout life; anytime you feel that you are going through a health challenge, do not hesitate to seek professional help.

When you experience some type of pain, or a cold or infection, you don't feel ashamed to seek the help of a doctor. The same should apply to any health condition, including sexual dysfunction. Seeking professional help, even if you did not have insurance, can be the best investment you ever made in yourself and for yourself. Remember, there is a solution for you, regardless of your age and your gender.

Important Message

Not all possible sexual conditions, causes and treatments have been discussed here but the most common ones that affect the vast majority of people. For further details contact your urologist, your gynecologist, The American Urological Association, The American College of Obstetricians and Gynecologists or the American Diabetes Association.

> **FOR MORE READINGS AND RELIABLE WEBSITES ON SEXUAL HEALTH AND OTHER TOPICS DISCUSSED IN THIS GUIDE REFER TO:**
>
> - The American Foundation for Urologic Disease Inc.: www.au.org
> - American Urological Association: www.auanet.org/index.cfm.
> - www.erectilefunction.org
> - Sexual Medicine Society of North America: www.smsna.org.
> - Medem: provides links such as: American College of Obstetricians and Gynecologists: www.medem.com
> - American Diabetes Association: www.diabetes.org
> - American Heart Association: www.amhrt.org
> - American Dietetic Association: www.eatright.org
> - Food and Drug Administration: www.fda.gov
> - National Institute for Health: www.nih.gov
> - International Food Information Council: http://ificinfo.health.org
> - Mayo Clinic: www.mayohealth.org
> - Juvenile Diabetes research foundation: www.jdf.org
> - Joslin Diabetes Center: www.joslin.org
> - International Diabetes Federation: www.idf.org

Contact Me

I wish you from the bottom of my heart the best of health.

I would love to hear your honest comments, the not so favorable ones first. I am not only looking for comments like "It is a good guide" or "I liked the information in this Guide" but also what I am looking to know is whether you **started acting immediately** on the valuable information provided to your fingertips and got your diabetes, cholesterol and blood pressure under control. I want to know if you started monitoring your sugar and blood pressure daily and whether you have been taking your medications on regular basis as prescribed by your doctor. Also I want to know whether you started and continued using the information in Action Step 4 and have built new good habits and whether the food and activity sections have helped you make more balanced favorable food and activity choices and helped you loose weight.

It took me several years of preparation and actual work on this guide before it came to fruition. My main goal throughout those years was to make it easily accessible and provide as many people as possible very important tools to help them **act and use these tools.** Consequently, more and more people can bring all aspects of their diabetes under control, prevent the deadly complications and have the best quality of life. I hope I was able to achieve that.

Good luck and good health.

LIFESTYLE MAKEOVER
2911 TURTLE CREEK BLVD.
SUITE 300
DALLAS, TX 75219
Email: mail@lifestyle-makeover.com
Website: www.lifestyle-makeover.com

Day/Date	FOOD LOG			
	What Food of Drink?	How Much?	From List A or List B?	How Can It Be Improved Next Time?
Breakfast				
Snack				
Lunch				
Snack				
Dinner				

This page titled Food Log may be copied by this guide's owner as frequently as needed.

\multicolumn{6}{c	}{**ACTIVITY LOG**}
Date	Day	Type of Activity / Number of Steps	Duration	**Weight Maintenance** Over 10,000 Steps	**Weight Loss** 12,000-15,000 Steps
	Monday				
	Tuesday				
	Wednesday				
	Thursday				
	Friday				
	Saturday				
	Sunday				
	Monday				
	Tuesday				
	Wednesday				
	Thursday				
	Friday				
	Saturday				
	Sunday				
	Monday				
	Tuesday				
	Wednesday				
	Thursday				
	Friday				
	Saturday				
	Sunday				
	Monday				
	Tuesday				
	Wednesday				
	Thursday				
	Friday				
	Saturday				
	Sunday				

This page titled Activity Log may be copied by this guide's owner as frequently as needed.

Sources of Data

Guidelines from Health Organizations:

American Diabetes Association (ADA)
World Health Organization (WHO)
Centers for Disease Control (CDC)
American Heart Association (AHA)
National Cholesterol Education Program (NCEP)
American Foundation for Urologic Disease
American Association of Clinical Endocrinologists (AACE)

Landmark Trials:

Diabetes Control and Complication Trial (DCCT)
United Kingdom Prospective Diabetes Study (UKPDS)
Diabetes Prevention Program (DPP)
"HOT"
"JNC 6" and "JNC 7"
Heart Protection Study (HPS)
Collaborative Atorvastatin Diabetes Study (CARDS)
"ALLHAT"

Professional Journals, Books and Manuals:

US Pharmacists
Drug Topics
Pharmacist's Letter
IDEA International Fitness Organization Journal
The Diet Revolution manual (by Ginger Schrimer Ph.D. R.D., Med 2000 Inc. Continuing Education 2004)
Diabetes State Management Manual (The University of Texas at Austin College of Pharmacy continuing Education manuals 2004 and 2006)
"NET CARB COUNTER" by Maggie Greenwood-Robinson Ph.D.
"Exubera" Medication Guide by Pfizer
American Pharmacists Associations (APhA) Journal

The intriguing stories of people and their ominous behaviors and some others with success stories, are real and true to life, making this guide one of a kind. Some stories like John Doe's, are fictitious but *all of these situations constitute a real learning platform and solutions* for millions of people who tend to have similar behaviors. *People can and have the power to make the change to healthier paths; this guide will show you how.*

Throughout my 20 years of pharmacy practice I have compiled the revealing stories of people with preventable chronic conditions whom I personally counseled and genuinely cared for. Although there are some success stories of people having their condition under full control, they are a minority.

All people with diabetes and other chronic ailments will, in one way or another, relate and learn from each of these characters' particular and revealing situations.

Any person, whether his or her diabetes is under control or not, will benefit tremendously from the practical solutions to ALL of the comprehensive challenges that any diabetic faces on a daily basis.

Since I was obese and leading a sedentary life as a child until late adolescence, the Lifestyle Section in Action Step 4 was the culmination of my decades of search for a balanced weight loss and maintenance method where there is no dieting, no deprivation or elimination of any food groups. I have found it and I share those revealing findings in Action Step 4. After extensive, protracted and targeted professional readings and specialization in related topics and lots and lots of patience and hard work over several years I put together all the pieces of the puzzle.

I took all the most updated professional research information from reliable institutions and sources (as referenced in Sources of Data on the last page of the guide) and blended it in seamlessly, using simple terms, in the various topics discussed in Action Step 4, and all through out this guide.

I can truly relate to you the reader if you have a weight problem and currently leading a sedentary lifestyle as I have been in your shoes, not long ago and I know first hand what you are going through. Believe me you can improve your current health and ward off deadly diseases if you act on the simple information provided to you. It is much simpler than you think.

The search has been done for you and all you have to do is take action and make the gradual change for the better. It took me decades to find out the truth. It is yours at your fingertips; all you have to do is act on it and get well.